SKIN
CONDITIONS

A SELF-HELP GUIDE
COMBINING ORTHODOX AND COMPLEMENTARY APPROACHES TO HEALTH

HASNAIN WALJI & DR ANDREA KINGSTON

Headway · Hodder & Stoughton

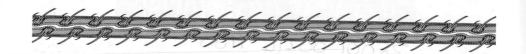

*This book is dedicated to the seekers of health
and to those who help them find it.*

Cataloguing in Publication Data is available from the British Library

ISBN 0 340 60559 6

First published 1994
Impression number 10 9 8 7 6 5 4 3 2 1
Year   1998   1997   1996   1994

Printed in Great Britain for Hodder & Stoughton Educational, a division of Hodder Headline Plc, 338 Euston Road, London NW1 3BH by Page Bros (Norwich) Ltd.

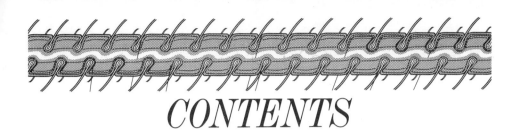

CONTENTS

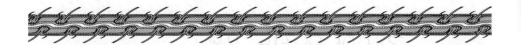

Note: Any information given in this book is not intended to be taken as a replacement for medical advice. Any person with a condition requiring medical attention should consult a medical professional.

ACKNOWLEDGEMENTS

I should like to express my gratitude to Dr Andrea Kingston for her valuable input, not just from from a GP's point of view, but also for the enlightened way she dealt with a number of apparent contradictions between orthodox medicine and complementary therapies; to nutritionist Angela Dowden for offering many pertinent suggestions; to Sato Liu of the Natural Medicines Society for her assistance in providing contacts and arranging interviews with practitioners; and to my agent Susan Mears for her encouragement and practical help.

This book could not possibly have been written without the co-operation of the following practitioners who have so willingly endured my interruptions: acupuncture – John Hicks and Peter Mole; aromatherapy – Christine Wildwood; naturopathy – Jan De Vries; homoeopathy – Michael Thompson; and anthroposophical medicine – Dr Morris Orange. A practitioner who must be singled for special acknowledgement is homoeopath Beth MacEoin, for her so very prompt and painstaking review of the chapter on homoeopathy.

I must thank my daughter Sukaina for giving her time during vacation from university for wading through research papers and books and extracting relevant information. Last but not least, I wish to thank my wife Latifa whose gentle care and concern, not to mention long hours typing the manuscript, enabled me to complete this book.

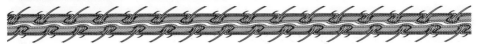

Foreword To The Series
from the Natural Medicines Society

When we visit our doctor's surgery and are given a diagnosis, we often receive a prescription at the same time. More people than ever are now aware that there may be complementary treatments available and would like to explore the possibilities, but do not know which kind of treatment would be most useful for their problem.

There are books on just about every treatment available, but few which start from this standpoint: the patient interested in knowing the options for treating their particular condition – which treatment is available or useful, what the treatment involves, or what to expect when consulting the practitioner.

The Headway Healthwise series will provide the answers for those wishing to consider what treatment is available, once the doctor has diagnosed their condition. Each book will cover both the orthodox and complementary approaches. Although patients are naturally most interested in relieving their immediate symptoms, the books show how complementary treatment goes much deeper; underlying causes are explored and the patient is treated as a whole.

It is important to stress that it is not the intention of this series to replace the expertise of the doctors and practitioners, nor to encourage self-treatment, but to show the options available to the patient.

As the consumer charity working for freedom of choice in medicine, the Natural Medicines Society welcomes the Headway Healthwise series. Although the Natural Medicines Society does not recommend people who are taking prescribed orthodox medicines to stop doing so, our aim is to introduce them to complementary forms of treatment. We believe the orthodox system of medicine is often best used as a last, not first, resort when other, gentler, methods fail or are inappropriate.

Giving patients the information to make their choice is the purpose of this series. With the increasing use of complementary medicine within the NHS, knowing the complementary options is vital both to the patients and to their doctors in the search for better health care.

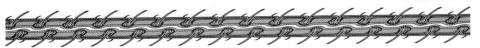

Foreword

As we approach the twenty-first century, those of us who concern ourselves with our health and the increasing number of threats we sustain to it from pollution and the pace and the complexity of modern life, as well as from legislation which in order to protect us, also restricts our freedom, we become aware of one overriding need – that of returning to Nature, from whence we came and grew strong in earlier times.

This has shown itself in our desire to eat more natural food, take more natural remedies and, above all, live a more natural life-style, which is more self-supportive. This is accompanied by a general trend towards the individual taking charge of their own health programme instead of leaving it entirely to a health expert.

Implicit in this trend is an increasing demand for knowledge: if we are going to take decisions about our bodies, we need to know a little of how they work and what treatment options are open to us. Books such as this one, which is part of a series on common health conditions and treatment options available, are furnishing a great contemporary need to inform the individual of the scope of the treatment choices.

Skin Conditions is a particularly valuable title because skin and skin complaints represent the first line of defence in the body, often affording a valued early warning that something we are doing or taking into the system is not agreeing with it. As such, often the simplest and most natural remedies are sufficient to persuade the body to restore homeostasis (balanced good health), whereas to resort immediately to the more powerful measures afforded by orthodox medical treatment could, at this initial stage, suppress the body's own natural defences and mask what it is trying to tell us.

Illness today is viewed in a completely different way from that of previous times when it was an enemy to be vanquished. Now it can be looked upon as the body's artwork: a creative expression of what is inharmonious in a person's life. With skin complaints, there is sometimes the sense of a person being 'rubbed up the wrong way' by their environment. The picture the body paints on its surface may not be welcome or pretty but it is valuable, and with the help of Nature and the three 'Os' – open mind, options and the opportunities to exercise them, the picture can be changed.

Jillie Collings, BA *Author, Health Writer and Council Member of the NMS*

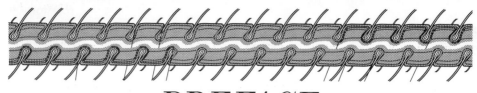

PREFACE

Headway Healthwise is a concise new series which takes the original approach of looking at common ailments and describing how they may be treated using complementary therapies. The aim of the series is not to replace the orthodox medical approach but complement it by giving readers an overview of how they may be helped by consulting complementary practitioners.

Once a condition has been diagnosed by a GP, those wishing to avail themselves of other forms of treatment will find this book particularly useful. The intention of this series is not to recommend that people who are taking prescribed orthodox medicines should stop taking these; it is to introduce them to alternative and complementary forms of treatment which may enable them to reduce the number of orthodox prescriptions they take and, in some cases, to obviate the need for orthodox prescriptions altogether.

We have attempted to present the information in a style that is clear and easy to read. The central approach is to look at common skin conditions from different perspectives by providing you with descriptions of several complementary therapies. While cautioning against self-medication, the book has been written to encourage you to take charge of your own health by making an informed choice of which therapy, or therapies, you will try.

An overview of common skin complaints is given in the first chapter and the kind of treatment to expect from one's GP is covered in the second chapter. The third chapter deals with such factors as lifestyle, diet and nutrition in the management of skin disorders – later chapters look at complementary approaches to the subject.

The one common factor that underpins all the alternative or complementary therapeutic techniques described in this book is the belief in the healing power of the body. Practitioners recognise that the body possesses an inherent ability to cure itself. This gives a clear message to the patient of his role in the healing process – that of the mind willing the body to heal.

At first sight this may appear to challenge the approach of orthodox medicine, in which the therapeutic objective is to cure the

diseased part of the body. The patient has no role to play, except dutifully to take the medicine. The concept of a white-coated god who possesses the magic pill to cure is the result of fear combined with a lack of understanding of the nature of disease and, to an even greater extent, that of health.

This book is an attempt to dispel the myths and to bring about a greater understanding of the issues relating to health and healing, which go beyond the realms of simple anatomy and biology. The recognition that orthodox medicine and complementary therapies need not be mutually exclusive can go a long way towards promoting the integrated medicine of the twenty-first century.

Hasnain Walji
Milton Keynes
November, 1993

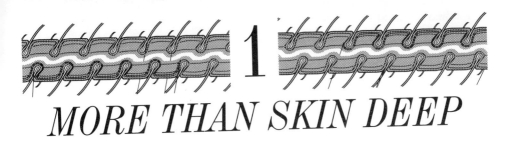

1

MORE THAN SKIN DEEP

Beauty, they say, is only skin deep. But how deep is skin?

There is much more to skin than what we see on the surface. Surprisingly, skin is an organ in the same way as the heart or brain. It is, in fact, the largest organ of the body. Weighing around 3 kg it covers an area of 2 sq m. It is made up of millions of cells surrounding countless nerve endings which sense pain, heat, cold and pressure. It regulates body temperature, prevents dehydration, facilitates waste disposal, and is the body's messenger of sensations to the brain. Skin tells us when we are pricked, pinched, punched, caressed, tickled or massaged.

As we continuously expose our skin to stresses, such as sunlight, wind, bacteria and chemical detergents, it reacts by producing a variety of painful and unsightly eruptions, such as acne, rashes and ulcers. At the same time, many skin conditions are an indication of imbalances in our bodies. Indeed, some complementary practitioners consider the appearance of a skin disorder as the body's means of eliminating an internal imbalance. The symptoms are seen to be healthy signs of the body's attempts to heal from the inside out.

However, some skin conditions can actually interfere with how skin functions. For example, it has already been indicated that the skin is vital for controlling body temperature. The skin is supplied by hundreds of thousands of small blood vessels, which expand when the body is hot and cause heat to be lost via the bloodstream. Sweat glands also help to regulate temperature, as the sweat cools the skin's surface as it evaporates. Specialised glands in the skin produce pigment, which help to protect us from penetration by the sun's harmful ultraviolet rays. Any skin conditions which interrupt these vital functions are potentially very serious. There is a rare condition called *hereditary ectodermal dysplasia* where there are virtually no sweat glands present in the skin, and the person affected is unable to control his or her body temperature. This can result in life-threatening overheating. Any condition which causes the skin to crack, such as eczema or widespread psoriasis, can lead to the loss of body fluids and allow the entry of harmful bacteria into the skin and sometimes into the bloodstream.

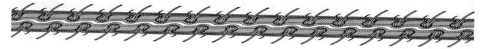

There is now good evidence that diet affects the ability of the skin to heal itself. Vitamin C, for example, is needed to help the skin to heal and is used in the formation of the connective tissue which joins the skin to the underlying tissues.

Generalised illnesses, such as diabetes, can affect the skin a great deal since it becomes much more prone to infection. Fungal conditions of the skin and bacterial infections, such as boils, are much more common if you suffer from diabetes. Even mental health can be reflected in the state of the skin. Some people with psychiatric problems deliberately damage the skin and may perpetuate an infection by repeatedly scratching the skin at the site of the infection. This is called *dermatitis artefacta.* In addition, people suffering from delusions may imagine insects on their body and may obsessionally scratch themselves thinking that they are infested.

However, this book confines itself to some of the more common skin disorders that are likely to be treated, initially, by your GP. The section on skin cancers is an exception, but has been included because such cancers have been the subject of much recent media interest.

It is always best to consult a qualified practitioner about a persistent rash rather than to treat it yourself. There may be an underlying cause to the problem that needs further investigation. You may well be given advice on skin care and on how to look after yourself generally, including advice on nutrition. Many skin conditions, including psoriasis, eczema and infections, are more usually present and more severe when a person is run down. Self-treatment is only wise if you are sure that you know what the problem is and how it should be treated.

What Is Skin?

The image that stares back at us in the mirror is sometimes our only concern, and we spend a great deal of time and money beautifying that image. Little do we realise that our bodies are constantly throwing off old skin and replacing it with new skin. Indeed, what we see in the mirror is really a layer of dead, old cells. This outermost layer is called the *epidermis.* The true skin, or the *dermis,* is between the epidermis and the lower layer, the *hypodermis.*

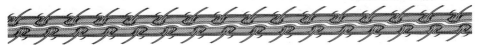

The Epidermis

This layer varies in thickness, being thickest on the soles of the feet and palms of the hands, and thinnest in the eyelids. It is generally thicker in men than in women, and becomes thinner with age.

What we see as 'skin' is the outermost part of the epidermis, which is composed of dead cells that form a tough, protective coating. In fact, the cells can be likened to a tiled roof with many overlapping layers. If this 'roof' is well maintained, the skin will look soft and beautiful; if not, the skin will be rough and flaky.

The lower layer of the epidermis continuously produces new cells by division. They move up to the surface and replace the cells that fall off. As they move up, they are transformed into a hard, durable protein called *keratin*, which is the main constituent of the horny, protective outer layer of the skin. Our bodies depend on this protective layer as it prevents dehydration – without it we would be dead in a few hours.

Normally, it takes three to four weeks for the newly-born cells in the lower layer to reach the outer surface, and it is remarkable how the body creates just the right number of new cells to replace the ones that are lost. This ingenious control mechanism ensures that our skin never wears out. However, the system can slow down with age or because of an imbalance in the body's functions.

The melanin-producing cells for skin pigmentation, known as *melanocytes*, are also present in the epidermis. The colour and quality of the skin is determined by the distribution and quality of these cells. Exposure to sunlight stimulates melanin production to provide a degree of natural sunscreening.

The Dermis

Under the epidermis, fitting like a jigsaw, is the dermis – the true skin which is composed of connective tissue and which contains the sweat glands, sebaceous glands (that produce the oily substance called *sebum*) and hair follicles. It is the fibrous tissue in this layer of the skin that determines how youthful, or otherwise, you look. The fibrous tissue (*collagen* and *elastin*) maintain the epidermis, and as the elastic qualities of the skin weaken, the dreaded wrinkles, progressive lines and sags appear. Medical research suggests that how we age depends on our genetic programming, but the ravages of pollution, excessive exposure to sunlight and an unhealthy diet can all lead to premature ageing.

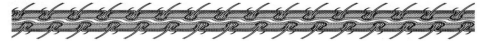

The Hypodermis

This is the deepest layer of the skin and is composed of fat cells, which are stored in connective tissue. Its function is to keep us warm and to cushion the body from blows. Fat distribution determines the shape of our bodies, and women tend to have a different distribution of fat to protect their unborn babies. The hypodermis also serves as an energy store which the body can draw upon in case of need, for instance in severe illness or starvation. Athletes burn off most of this during long, regular exercise sessions.

Functions of the skin

- Provides a protective barrier between the environment and the body.
- Shields internal organs from injury, sunlight and germs.
- Sensory organ – it is sensitive to touch, pain and temperature.
- Keeps body temperature constant.
- Provides a waterproof barrier.
- Serves to maintain the balance of body fluids.
- Organ for elimination of fluids, minerals and other biochemicals.

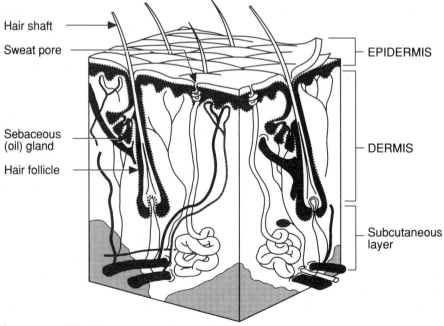

The structure of the skin

Common conditions

Skin infections:
- boils, abscesses and other skin infections
- cellulitis
- impetigo
- shingles
- cold sores
- athlete's foot
- ringworm
- nappy rash

Eczema:
- atopic eczema
- seborrhoeic eczema

- contact dermatitis

Urticaria (hives)

Psoriasis

Acne

Skin cancers:
- solar keratosis
- Bowen's disease
- malignant melanoma
- basal cell carcinoma
- squamous cell carcinoma

Benign skin conditions:
- vitiligo
- warts and verrucas

Skin Infections

Boils, Abscesses And Other Skin Infections

Our first line of defence against disease-causing bacteria is the outer layer of the skin. When this is breached, boils and other skin infections can occur.

As soon as germs invade the barrier, the body's fighting force, the *immune system*, is mobilised into action. More blood is pumped into the area and the skin tissue is instructed to alter its cell structure and cordon off the infected area, so limiting the spread of the bacteria.

As a result of the increased blood supply, the skin becomes red, swollen and warm. Pain occurs when the swollen skin is stretched. Sometimes the inflammation may subside quickly but, if it does not, then the cordoning off process continues, resulting in the formation of pus in the centre of the boil. Pus is a mixture of blood fluids, white cells and bacteria.

Eventually, the boil comes to a head on the skin surface and opens to release the pus. Once this happens, the pain disappears and the infection is quickly healed. If the pus remains encapsulated in the skin, it is called an *abscess.*

While boils themselves are not usually considered serious, they may become a cause of generalised illness if the immune system is

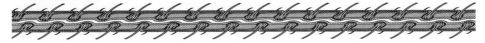

not able to contain the bacteria within the boil and they enter the bloodstream, thus spreading elsewhere in the body.

Cellulitis

Cellulitis is an infection that spreads within the skin, and is characterised by a puffy, red swelling that extends from the site of the original infection and feels warm to the touch. The inflammation of cellulitis is usually too diffuse (spread out over a wide area) to cause the formation of pus anywhere other than in the original boil.

Impetigo

Highly contagious, impetigo is an infection of the skin caused by *Streptococcus* and *Staphylococcus* bacteria. It results in the eruption of small, red, raised bumps that develop into tiny blisters and ooze a sticky fluid to leave raw, red sores. These sores may appear on the cheeks, the lips and at the nostrils. Their appearance is similar to that of cold sores or herpes, except that impetigo spreads more rapidly and does not confine itself to one part of the body.

Shingles

A painful, blistered rash that can develop only in people who have had chickenpox at some time in their lives. Beginning with severe pain and without any apparent reason, the onset of shingles is followed by a skin eruption, or rash, in the painful area. The rash normally clears after a few weeks, often leaving scars where the blisters have been.

Cold Sores

Cold sores are small blisters which usually appear around the mouth and nostrils and develop into uncomfortable, watery sores. They are caused by *Herpes simplex*, a common and infectious virus which can also attack other parts of the face. While this condition can be painful and annoying, it is not a serious health condition. However, cold sores are contagious and can have a dangerous effect on babies.

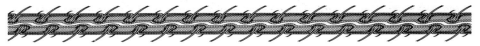

Athlete's Foot

Itchy, inflamed skin between the toes is a sign of this fungal infection caused by the fungus *Tinea pedis*. The skin may also crack or flake off, exposing red, tender skin underneath. If the condition persists, toenails may also be affected and the nails may even separate from the nail beds.

Ringworm

Medically called *Tinea corporis*, ringworm is a highly contagious fungal skin infection that results in rough, dry, slightly-raised eruptions that usually occur in circular patches.

Nappy Rash

Prolonged wetting, coupled with skin irritation by substances contained in the urine or faeces, is the cause of nappy rash. Some babies may be more susceptible than others. It may also be the first indication of a sensitive skin.

Eczema

The term *eczema* really just means 'inflammation of the skin' and is interchangeable with *dermatitis*. However, most doctors in the UK reserve the term *dermatitis* for inflammation which is caused by an outside agent, and the term *eczema* for all forms of the condition which originate 'internally', that is, those that are a part of the person's constitution.

A chronic skin condition, eczema is characterised by inflammation of the skin, irritation and the shedding of dry skin cells. Inevitably, the itching results in scratching. Dry, scaly, itchy, inflamed, and often sore and bloody, eczema can cause physical and mental distress to the sufferer. Though it usually strikes during childhood and clears up after puberty and adolescence, it can occur at any age. Those with an allergy to bleaches, detergents, wax polishes and so on, can develop eczema on their hands. Stress is another factor that can contribute to the problem. Central heating, very hot weather or excessive clothing and humidity may aggravate the irritation. There are several types of eczema.

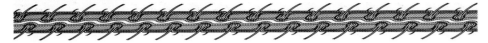

Atopic Eczema

This affects people with a family history of asthma or hay fever, and is believed to be the result of a malfunction in the immune system which overreacts to a wide range of stimuli.

Seborrhoeic Eczema

Not to be confused with atopic eczema, this usually only affects babies and adults (particularly men) from their twenties to their forties, and is usually worse on the scalp, but it can spread to the face and body, especially the groin and armpits. *Discoid eczema* (multiple, small, round areas of red, scaly skin) is common in people over 60 years of age.

Contact Dermatitis Or Eczema

This is a common form of eczema which develops very quickly and is sometimes caused by an allergy, but often occurs for no known reason. *Allergic contact dermatitis* occurs when a body develops a sudden allergy to substances it has previously treated as harmless, perhaps for years.

Urticaria (Hives)

Urticaria, also known as *hives*, is characterised by raised and swollen wheals with blanched centres, which vary in size from small, pimple-like spots to raised patches several inches across. Hives are caused by the release of histamine under the skin and may be triggered by food, food additives and drugs, as well as by sensitivity to the cold, house dust, pollen or even sunlight. Often in many cases there is no identifiable cause.

Psoriasis

Psoriasis is a non-contagious skin disorder with sharply-bordered red patches covered with silvery scales, which can be itchy and very painful. Usually, the problem is no more than cosmetic. It is a common disorder, affecting 2 per cent of the population. There is no one cause of this condition, but it consists of abnormalities in the lining of the skin's blood vessels, the skin cells themselves, and the accelerated rate at which the outer skin layer reproduces itself and is

replaced by new cells from beneath. As a result, live cells accumulate and form characteristic thickened patches covered with dead, flaking skin. The skin eruption is sometimes accompanied by a painful swelling and stiffness of the joints, which can be very disabling.

Acne

Acne is a condition generally associated with the teenage years and the early twenties. Its characteristics are facial spots and scars, which cause untold misery to countless youngsters just when they are trying to look their best.

It is an inflammatory condition occurring in the hair follicles of the sebaceous glands. Sebum, produced by the glands, acts as a natural lubricant for the skin. But when too much is produced the glands can become blocked and inflamed, causing blackheads and pimples. Sometimes the blocked glands become infected, and pus and sebum build up under the skin, forming large pimples or cysts, which can leave scars and pitting.

Hormone levels during puberty are also known to affect the amount of sebum released.

Skin Cancers

There are various types of cancer of the skin. Prolonged or unaccustomed exposure to the ultraviolet (UV) radiation in sunlight increases the risk of developing cancer. Rodent ulcer (mostly found on the face), squamous cell carcinoma and malignant melanoma are common forms of cancer related to long-term exposure to sunlight. Bowen's disease, a rare skin disorder that can be cancerous, may also be related to exposure to sunlight. Less common types of skin cancer include Paget's disease of the nipple and *mycosis fungoides*. Both produce inflammation similar to that of eczema. Kaposi's sarcoma is a type of skin cancer often found in patients with AIDS.

Benign Skin Conditions

Vitiligo

This is a disorder in which patches of skin lose their colour. White

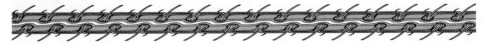

patches are particularly obvious in dark-skinned people, usually occurring on the face and hands, and in the armpits and groin. The affected skin is particularly sensitive to sunlight.

Vitiligo is thought to be a disorder that causes an absence of melanocytes, the specialised cells responsible for secreting the skin pigment *melanin.*

Warts

Warts are small lumps on the skin surface caused by an overgrowth of skin cells. Triggered by a viral infection, the infected skin cells begin to grow and divide abnormally as the body reacts to the virus. This is because the regulatory control of cell division is disturbed, and the cells continue to build upon themselves. They may also occur on the sole of the foot and are known as *verrucas*. As they grow into the skin instead of outwards, they can be quite painful.

The ordinary wart virus is very common and contagious, and there is little you can do to prevent your exposure to it. Some of us may be more susceptible to these infections than others but, generally, children are more susceptible than adults. There is usually no pain, nor other symptoms, unless the warts are subjected to pressure or friction.

Taking Charge

In the following chapters we shall look in some detail at the signs, symptoms and causes of the above common skin conditions, as well as the different therapeutic options available for managing the ailments. These options range from what is available in the GP's surgery to dietary measures and herbal remedies. Various relevant complementary therapies will be discussed in subsequent chapters to enable you to make an informed choice of a suitable management programme in the treatment and prevention of your skin disorders.

WHAT CAN YOUR GP OFFER?

Most people have trouble with their skin at some time in their lives, even if it is just a minor infection, such as a boil or measles.

Changes in the appearance of our skin, for whatever reason, can be very upsetting, since in our society so much emphasis is placed on looks. The commonest chronic skin conditions, such as eczema and psoriasis, need to be regarded with sympathy and understanding since they are both conditions which can last a lifetime and which may require a change of lifestyle in order to keep them under control.

More than one in ten people attending their GP are seeking help for a skin problem, and most can be dealt with quite adequately with the large number of preparations available.

The most important task for the GP is usually to explain how a treatment should be applied and to discuss other aspects of lifestyle, such as bathing, clothing and exposure to sun, which can profoundly affect some conditions.

There is an enormous range of skin conditions and it would be beyond the scope of this book to describe them all. What follows is an explanation of the commoner chronic skin conditions, a look at some of the more usual infections and a description of cancers.

Bacterial Skin Infections

Boils, Abscesses And Other Skin Infections

Normally, the skin provides protection against bacteria and substances harmful to the body but, for various reasons, this first line of defence is sometimes unsuccessful. This can happen if the surface of the skin is damaged so that bacteria can get in, or if the bacterium is very virulent (extremely infective). Infection will also result if there are large numbers of bacteria which overwhelm the body's defences in the bloodstream, particularly if they are not working properly.

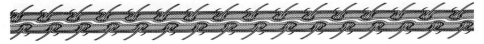

The skin produces an inflammatory response to the bacteria by increasing the blood supply to the area and leaks fluids out from the small blood vessels. Histamine and other chemicals are released and the body's defence mechanism, in the form of white cells, begin to attack the bacteria. The result of this is red, swollen, warm skin which may become stretched and painful. If the bacteria are not fully eliminated in this way, a 'walling-off' process begins to try and localise the area of infection. Pus then begins to form and a boil may develop. Pus is a mixture of fluid from the blood, dead white cells and bacteria. A carbuncle may develop if the boil becomes large with multiple centres of pus formation.

The natural course is either for the boil to come to a head at the surface of the skin, eventually opening to allow the pus to escape, or it is gradually absorbed by the body. If the collection of pus becomes trapped in a cavity, it is called an abscess. Abscesses can occur in many parts of the body. A boil or abscess may release germs into the bloodstream if the immune system cannot cope, and a generalised illness called *septicaemia* or *bacteraemia* may result. However, this is relatively rare.

Minor infections of this kind, such as on the finger or toenails, are usually self-limiting, and can often be treated without a visit to the doctor. A larger boil or abscess, if it is at an early stage, may have to be treated with antibiotics, or, if it is at an advanced stage, incised and drained under a local or general anaesthetic. The cavity left behind may need to be packed with specially-soaked gauze to allow healing to occur from the bottom of the abscess.

Cellulitis

Cellulitis is a term for an infection which spreads within the skin and underlying tissue, and is not walled within a specific area. This might occur after an insect bite or some other relatively minor trauma to the skin. It may also be an extension of a localised infection, such as a boil or abscess. One form of cellulitis is called *erysipelas,* which classically occurs as a spreading redness on the face. Unlike boils, cellulitis, because it is not localised, cannot be excised and drained, but should be treated promptly with antibiotics to prevent the spread of germs to the bloodstream.

Impetigo

This is a rather different skin infection, which is usually caused by

two specific forms of bacteria: *Staphylococcus* or *Streptococcus*. It frequently occurs on the faces of children, and forms yellow crusts which spread rapidly over a few days. It is highly contagious. Luckily, it is very sensitive to local and oral antibiotics, and leaves the skin without any scarring once treated.

All these conditions are most likely to appear when you are run down, tired, weakened by poor diet or suffering from diabetes. So it is worth seeking treatment, especially if they are recurrent.

Germs can sometimes be passed from person to person in the family, and the *Staphylococcus* bacteria can live permanently in the nose or throat, multiplying on the skin when it gets the opportunity. If your doctor suspects it is spreading, the whole family may be given treatment with a special antibiotic nose cream to try and eliminate the bacteria completely.

Shingles

Shingles is known medically as *herpes zoster*, from a Greek word *herpes* meaning 'to creep' and *zoster* meaning 'girdle' or 'belt'. This condition is caused by the same virus that causes chicken-pox. After an attack of chicken-pox, most viral organisms survive and lie dormant in certain sensory nerves. As the immune system declines because of age or stress, the virus is activated to cause shingles.

The first symptom of shingles is usually severe pain, which tends to have a stinging quality. A few days later, this is followed by a rash in the area of the pain which blisters and then scabs over. The rash normally goes after two or three weeks, often leaving scars where the blisters have been. However, the pain may persist for months, or even years, and this is known as *post-herpetic neuralgia*. This disabling condition tends to affect older people rather than the young, and can be notoriously difficult to treat.

Cold Sores

These small blisters, which are caused by the *herpes simplex* virus, usually appear in a cluster around the mouth or nostrils and develop into nasty, watery sores. The virus is common and infectious, and can attack other parts of the face. It is usually passed on from adult to child, and a first attack may cause feverishness and sickness as well as blisters. The virus remains dormant in the body but, in some people, it can be reactivated by exposure to cold, sunburn, infections or even menstruation.

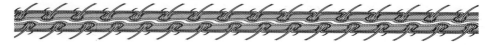

Treatment

The usual treatment for both shingles and cold sores is an antiviral cream called acyclovir (trade name: Zovirax). This cream, when applied in the very early stages, will shorten an episode and make it less severe, which will also tend to reduce the chances of suffering post-herpetic neuralgia. For those whose immune systems are not working properly, that is, people who have another serious illness, or for anyone in whom the attacks recur, tablet treatment with acyclovir may be given. This may lengthen the interval between episodes, but does not actually act as a cure. Once the virus is in the body, it cannot be eradicated completely.

Fungal Skin Infections

Athlete's Foot

Associated with wearing shoes and sweating, this common foot infection is a type of ringworm caused by the fungus *Tinea pedis*. It can be picked up in public places, such as showers and changing rooms and, once contracted, it can be hard to get rid of. The skin on and between the toes becomes sore and itchy, and may crack or peel away, exposing red, tender skin underneath. Sometimes small blisters and rashes appear.

Treatment

There is a variety of antifungal creams which are effective against Athlete's foot, for example, clotrimazole (trade name: Canesten) and miconazole. These need to be applied twice daily until the skin is completely normal. General hygiene measures and keeping the feet as cool and dry as possible are essential.
Tinea infection of the nails is much more difficult to treat and usually requires prolonged tablet treatment. A number of preparations are available, for example, griseofulvin, terbinafine (trade name: Lamisil). Griseofulvin has been associated with severe side-effects of the liver, but Lamisil is generally regarded as the safer drug and needs to be taken for a shorter time. An antifungal solution to paint on the nails has recently come on to the market. Claimed to be as effective as tablet treatment, this is called amorolfine (trade name: Loceryl) and is only suitable for adults.

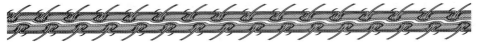

Ringworm

The highly contagious infection of the skin, known popularly as ringworm, is also medically called *tinea*. The term 'ringworm' is really a misnomer, since no worm is involved, and it is actually caused by a fungal infection. The ring shape is formed as the infection spreads. Warm, moist areas, such as the armpits, groin, beneath the breasts and on the feet, are the most common places for ringworm.

Treatment

Any of the usual range of antifungal creams mentioned above should get rid of this condition if used regularly until the rings have completely gone. Ringworm can be transmitted by cats and dogs, so if you have a pet, get it checked out by a vet and have it treated if necessary.

Nappy Rash

A common condition affecting babies with otherwise healthy skin, nappy rash results from an irritant dermatitis caused by ammonia (which is a breakdown product of urine) combined with an infection with the yeast *Candida* (thrush). While usually confined to the nappy area, the thrush element can spread as a rash on to the abdomen, and can look quite severe and alarming.

Treatment

Antifungal creams may be combined with mild hydrocortisone if there is severe inflammation. Changing the nappy regularly and exposing the baby's bottom whenever possible will also help healing.

Eczema

Most people will have seen someone with eczema and will be familiar with the red, scaly patches which can occur anywhere on the body. There are several different sorts of eczema which are categorised mainly by their appearance or where they occur on the body.

Atopic Eczema

This is, perhaps, the most commonly discussed form of eczema. The word 'atopic' means a tendency towards *hypersensitivity*, an

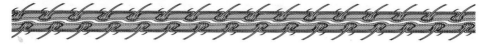

overreaction to everyday substances. Atopic eczema is the sort that may be inherited, that always appears in childhood and that may be associated with allergic conditions, such as asthma, hay fever and urticaria.

The exact causes of eczema are still unknown, but research has shown that it almost certainly involves the immune system in some way. The immune system is the body's own fighting force which, in this instance, is somehow inappropriately triggered and causes the redness and inflammation of the skin. Other predisposing factors include dry, irritable skin, emotional upset and susceptibility to skin infections. In about 5 per cent of sufferers, certain foods can precipitate (bring on) eczema, the commonest being cow's milk, eggs and food colourants.

It usually starts in babies of between 3 and 6 months of age, with eczematous patches largely on the cheeks, neck and in the groin. It may also spread to the arms and legs, but these areas are usually less severely affected. As the person grows older, the distribution of atopic eczema tends to change so that, in children, the areas around the eyes, ears and neck are first affected, and then behind the knees, the folds of the arms, hands and feet. In adults, the commonest problem areas are the back of the neck and folds of the joints.

The condition tends to improve with age, and almost two-thirds of children have virtually normal skin by the age of 6. Certain factors, however, may prolong the affliction. These include a strong family history of eczema, where the forearms and lower legs are affected and its onset after the age of 2 years.

Seborrhoeic Eczema

This type of eczema is usually present in adults rather than in children, and is most common between the ages of 20 and 40 years. It is used to describe eczema that is not generally inherited and which occurs around the scalp, neck, eyebrows and on the chest and back. The word 'seborrhoeic' is something of a misnomer and relates to the belief that the condition was caused by an excess of the fatty material, sebum, produced by glands in the skin. We now know that this is not the case.

It can be particularly bad behind the ears and around the temples and eyebrows, and may cause very bad dandruff. The ear canals may also be affected causing a condition called *otitis externa.*

There is some evidence to suggest that the fungus *Pitysporum ovale* actually causes seborrhoeic eczema. It is present in large amounts on

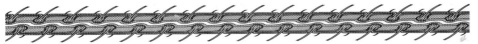

the skin of sufferers, but it is possible that it is only one of a number of factors that trigger the condition.

Discoid Eczema

This is another variety of eczema which is characterised by multiple small, round areas of red, scaly skin. It is common in people over 60 years, though may occur at any age. It frequently becomes infected.

Pompholyx

This is an eczema affecting the palms and soles. Generally, there are multiple blisters on the skin which can become quite large. This condition can be disabling and can last over many weeks or months if it is not properly treated or if it becomes infected.

Treatment

No matter how mild or severe the eczema, it is very important to avoid anything which is likely to irritate it. This may include soap and other detergents, as well as local heat. Wearing comfortable clothing made out of a natural fabric, such as cotton, next to the skin is also a sensible precaution.

Emollients And Soap Substitutes
Aqueous cream, oilatum emollient and E45 cream, among others, can all be used both as soap substitutes and to moisturise the skin. It is important, especially in children who may be badly affected, to establish a routine of moisturising twice a day. Soaking in the bath with an additive, such as Alpha Keri or Emulsiderm, also helps by allowing moisture into the skin and then sealing it in. This treatment alone is sufficient for a lot of children with mild eczema and also some adults.

Coal Tar
Like emollients, this treatment is also used effectively in cases of psoriasis, and the cruder the preparation, the more effective it tends to be. It may be applied by using bandages, which is especially helpful to children with atopic eczema who tend to scratch excessively. It requires quite a lot of effort and determination to use the bandages, but if it can be done at home it may avoid the nursing care which might necessitate a hospital admission. Some of the more refined tar preparations tend to be much less messy and for that reason may be more acceptable.

Steroid Creams
The use of mild steroid creams, even in young children, should be considered under medical supervision.

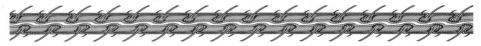

Atopic children may suffer some stunting of growth, but it is now generally accepted that the stunting is the result of the disease rather than of the use of steroid creams. For most children, 0.5% or 1% hydrocortisone is sufficient, and it is only rarely that stronger steroids, for example, Eumovate or Betnovate, are needed. It should be remembered that, in both adults and children, a small proportion are hypersensitive to hydrocortisone, which may end up making the eczema worse.

Antihistamines

In infants and young children, these are important in treatment, mainly because they have sedative properties. Because eczema is so itchy, many children will scratch incessantly at night, and the skin becomes thickened, infected and bleeds. Antihistamines can do a lot to prevent this from happening. It is likely that the non-sedating antihistamines which may be given to adults are of less value, though some people find that they help to reduce the itching.

Oral Steroids

Such steroids are virtually never used in children but, occasionally, adults with very severe eczema improve with them. Injections of a hormone substitute, adrenocorticotrophic hormone (ACTH), is given at weekly or fortnightly intervals in reducing dosages. This may cause a number of severe side-effects and is now not commonly used.

Antibiotics

These have a useful part to play, particularly in childhood eczema where infection is common. There is some evidence that one particular skin germ called *Staphyloccoccus aureus* may be involved as a trigger of eczema. It is certainly accepted, however, that secondary infection is common, and many sufferers of atopic eczema improve with an appropriate course of antibiotics. There is also a place for local antibiotics/steroid preparations.

Antifungal Agents

The presence of *Pitysporum ovale* has led to the development of antifungal shampoos, for example, ketaconazole and niconazole, which greatly improve seborrhoeic eczema. Some patients with atopic eczema also improve when antifungal creams are used on the skin. However, this is not a common regime to follow.

Potassium Permanganate Solution

This is generally reserved for pompholyx eczema. Large blisters may need to be emptied, followed by soaking in this purple-coloured solution before a dressing is applied. It is the only orthodox treatment that really helps this potentially severe form of eczema.

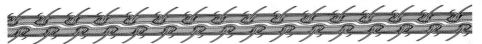

Evening Primrose Oil

EPO contains the substance gammalinolenic acid, levels of which have been shown to be lower than normal in some eczema sufferers. Scientific trials have shown that some eczema sufferers definitely benefit from taking capsules of EPO, and that most have reduction in itching and roughness of the skin. Research has shown that EPO is significantly more effective than giving placebo (dummy) treatment. EPO is not suitable for babies under 1 year, but children's capsules are now available. Adults need to take 12 capsules per day to derive the proper effect from this. A minimum of three months' treatment is needed to see if it works, as this is the length of time the skin takes to replenish itself. It can be a safe treatment with very few side-effects (see Chapter 3 for further details on EPO).

Allergic Or Contact Dermatitis

This condition resembles eczema, but the mechanism by which it occurs is different. Allergic or contact dermatitis occurs when a person becomes sensitised to a particular substance which is in contact with the skin. It may take more than one exposure for this to happen, but once the skin is sensitised it will happen each time there is a contact. This is called a *delayed hypersensitivity reaction*, and is really just a mistake that is made by the body's own defence mechanisms.

About 15 per cent of industrial dermatitis is allergic in origin. It is common, for example, hairdressers who have become allergic to shampoos or perming chemicals. Other substances which have been commonly implicated are nickel, chromate, lanolin, rubber chemicals, chrysanthemums and certain fragrances.

It is this sort of dermatitis that causes a number of women to change their make-up to a brand that is *hypoallergenic*, that is, unlikely to cause an allergic reaction. In fact, this hypoallergenic make-up uses substances which are found much less commonly and to which far fewer people have been exposed. This may be the only reason that they cause less allergy. It is quite possible that if they were to be widely used, just as many people would be allergic to these special cosmetics!

Treatment

Removal from the specific substance is essential, otherwise the condition will continue to get worse. Diagnoses such as fungal conditions and psoriasis should be excluded. Treatment usually needs

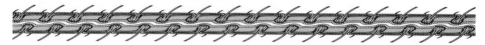

topical steroids which may, unfortunately, themselves act as sensitisers in some people.

Referral to a consultant for patch testing should be considered if the condition does not quickly resolve (subside) with treatment. Patch testing involves exposing the skin to a variety of substances which are likely to cause an allergic response. The dilution of the substance has to be carefully assessed so as not to cause an irritant dermatitis by mistake. This is then pricked on to the skin, and the condition of the skin reviewed a number of hours later. A red, inflamed response indicates a positive patch test. Allergic eczema may often become infected, and a combination of steroids and antibiotic creams has to be used with or without antibiotics taken by mouth.

Irritant Dermatitis

This is distinct from allergic dermatitis and is caused by a direct response of the skin to the substance concerned. It is more common than allergic dermatitis and accounts for about 70 per cent of cases of industrial dermatitis.

Acids and alkalis can both cause the condition if left on the skin for long enough, but other agents require repeated exposure for an irritant reaction to occur, and an example of this would be detergents. Other substances commonly causing irritant dermatitis are degreasing agents, and coolants. People with atopic eczema are more prone to irritant dermatitis than the rest of the population.

Treatment of both allergic and irritant dermatitis is on the same principle as eczema. Removal from the allergen or the substance which is causing irritation is essential, particularly with allergic dermatitis, to avoid chronic and intractable skin changes taking place.

Barrier creams used in industry are largely ineffective, but conditioning creams can help to prevent dermatitis caused by damage to the skin.

Urticaria (Hives) And Angio-oedema

Urticaria is also known as *wheals* or *hives*, and is much more common than the related angio-oedema. Many of you will be familiar with the appearance of urticaria with its irregular, lumpy, raised blotches on the skin which can be extremely itchy. It can also present as tiny round lumps. Many people with urticaria are atopic, and suffer from asthma, eczema or hay fever as well.

In most cases, it is caused by an allergic mechanism, and occurs in the deep layer of skin, the dermis. Substances to which the person is allergic may be in contact with the skin, inhaled or eaten. This prompts an inappropriate reaction in specialised cells in the body called *mast cells*. These release chemicals called *histamines* which cause blood vessels in the skin to become dilated (wider or larger). These blood vessels then leak fluid into the skin as part of the process of inflammation.

Urticaria may come and go within just a few hours, but in a minority of people it becomes chronic over months or even years.

When the reaction occurs below the level of the skin in the subcutaneous tissues, it is known as angio-oedema. The swelling in angio-oedema can be great and can involve gross swelling of the lips and also of the the tongue and throat. Limbs may also be involved. Occasionally, this can be life threatening and needs urgent medical treatment with adrenalin, steroids and antihistamine given by injection.

Urticaria may be triggered by many things. Usual examples of these are nuts, strawberries, eggs and shellfish. Some drugs, such as antibiotics or aspirin, can also be to blame.

Physical urticaria is also a well-documented phenomenon with wheals appearing in response to exercise, heat, sunshine, cold or pressure. Scratching the skin with a blunt instrument can produce the same reaction, which is known as *dermographism.*

With children, especially, it is often difficult to find the cause of urticaria, and keeping careful food diary records or trying elimination diets are probably not worthwhile unless the condition becomes chronic. In addition, since the chronic form lasts on average six to nine months, the urticaria will have settled by the time the investigation has finished. Very occasionally, chronic urticaria may be connected with a serious medical condition called *systemic lupus erythematosis* and it is always worth checking with your family doctor to make sure that this is not the cause of the problem.

Treatment

Some children are not at all bothered by their hives and, as symptoms will usually disappear in a day or two, no treatment is necessary. Most sufferers only visit their GP because they are fed up with the problem and are looking for instant relief. Unfortunately, it only has a cure when the precipitating substance can be identified and avoided. Otherwise the action of the medication just dampens down the condition.

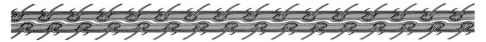

Antihistamines

These are the mainstay of treatment. The more modern antihistamines called Type 1 antihistamines (H1 blockers) reduce the size of the wheal as well as the itching. These antihistamines are virtually free from side-effects and they rarely cause sedation. Some chronic sufferers need to take them every day, and it is worth trying a variety of preparations to find the one which suits you the best. In severe cases, a better response has resulted from adding a histamine Type 2 receptor blocker (H2 blocker,) such as cimetidine (trade name: Tagamet). However, increasing the dose of the H1 blocker has been shown to have the same effect.

Oral Steroids

These may be used for chronic and severe urticaria which is disabling, but such use is rare. They may also be administered in short courses for just after an urticaria-inducing activity. If they have a chronic problem, some patients need to be on a maintenance dose for several months. Hereditary angio-oedema needs anabolic steroids to reduce the severity and frequency of attacks. Two examples of these are stanozolol and danazol. People who suffer from hereditary angio-oedema will generally be under the care of a consultant dermatologist. This form of the disease is caused by an enzyme deficiency and is treated with tranexamic acid tablets.

Psoriasis

This chronic skin condition affects between 1 and 2 per cent of the population worldwide. Its main features are the characteristic red, raised, scaly patches called *plaques*, which are often found on the elbows, knees and trunk. They have a silvery appearance which helps to distinguish them from patches of eczema. Any part of the body may be affected, including palms of the hands, soles of the feet and scalp, but it is rare to find psoriasis on the face. Many people with the condition are mildly affected and never bother to seek medical help, but it can cause great embarrassment and anxiety, especially among adolescents. For, while it is not usually itchy or painful, it may well be considered disfiguring to the sufferer.

When psoriasis develops, the upper layer of the skin, the epidermis, becomes much thicker than normal with an increased number of cells. These cells are produced at a greatly increased rate, and move from the bottom layer of the skin to the surface in only a few days instead of several weeks. The new cells are much stickier than ordinary cells, so instead of being shed in the normal way, they

build up on the surface to form plaques.

No-one knows how this process starts nor how it is maintained by the body, but certain trigger factors have been identified. These include some viral infections, such as influenza, and bacterial infections, such as streptococcal, stress, injury to the skin, and changes in hormone levels, for example around the menopause. Some drugs may bring on the condition, for example, drugs used in the prevention of malaria. There is also a hereditary tendency, though this is not always the most important factor.

Some recent research has suggested that psoriasis is caused by an unknown fault in the immune system, the body's own defence mechanism. Certain cells called *T-helper lymphocytes*, which are part of the immune system, have been found in psoriatic skin, but their exact role is still not clear.

Psoriasis may take many forms other than the plaques just described, such as *guttate psoriasis*, where large areas of the body may be covered in small, round, scaly spots, and the more severe *pustular psoriasis*, which affects the palms and soles. When the scalp alone is involved, it may look just like ordinary dandruff, but the usual shampoos will not be enough to clear it. In infants, it may first appear only in the nappy area, looking just like nappy rash, which can cause a great problem in diagnosis.

In a few unfortunate people, nearly the whole skin surface may be involved. This potentially life-threatening condition is called *erythrodermic psoriasis* and almost always needs urgent hospital admission. An extensive disease such as this is, thankfully, rare but it usually means the individual is unable to control heat and water loss from the body, which is why specialised care is needed.

Pitting of the nails is frequently seen in adults, and does not always correlate with the severity of the condition. There is nothing that can be done about this, but it does not cause any discomfort. A minority of people, however, develop arthritis from psoriasis. This usually affects the hands and is treated in a similar way to other types of joint problem, mostly with anti-inflammatory tablets.

Treatment

About 40 per cent of people with psoriasis either do not want or do not need treatment from their GP. Most will have just the odd patch which does not interfere with their lives. Some will manage with over-the-counter preparations of moisturisers to stop the skin from drying and cracking. The sun's ultraviolet rays have a beneficial effect, and can make plaques disappear completely in the summer months (although

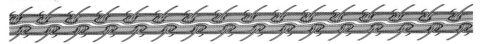

about 5 per cent of sufferers are made worse by exposure).
The other 60 per cent, however, will usually consult their GP for
treatment, and a few of those will need referral to a specialist, either to
confirm the diagnosis or for some of the special treatments which need
very close monitoring.

Many people who go to their GP for this complaint have never heard
of the condition before, and they are often relieved to hear that it is
neither infectious nor anything to do with skin cancer. A full
explanation and reassurance that it is treatable goes a long way to
helping sufferers come to terms with their psoriasis. Some people put
up with severe psoriasis for years without seeking advice, thinking that
nothing can be done. Unfortunately, many sufferers have the unrealistic
expectation that just a few days of applying a cream will do the trick and
that they can then forget about it.

Getting psoriasis under control is usually fairly easy with more recent
treatments, but it may then take some time to identify the trigger factors
and, even with careful recording of events, it may still remain a mystery
as to why the psoriasis flares up. In children, one very sensible step is
promptly to treat other skin infections. One particular bacteria,
Streptococcus, is renowned for causing psoriasis, and its immediate treatment with penicillin, or a similar antibiotic, may stop a flare up.

Day-to-day skin care is the mainstay of treatment for psoriasis.
Wearing comfortable clothing made from fibres such as cotton is a great
help and something that is often overlooked.

Moisturisers, Emollients And General Skin Care
With all but the most trivial psoriasis, a daily routine of skin care
becomes the most important aspect of treatment. Many people need to
use a soap substitute, such as aqueous cream or E45 cream, and a bath
additive, such as oilatum emollient. Vaseline may be all that is needed
for the occasional appearance of plaques. All these measures are likely
to keep the skin supple and stop it becoming cracked, painful and
infected.

Coal Tar
This treatment has been around a long time and is still used quite often.
It helps by descaling the patches, but needs to be applied carefully to
the plaques only, as it may irritate normal skin.

It is sometimes mixed with another 'descaling' agent, salicylic acid. In
general, the cruder and less refined the coal tar preparation, the more
effective it is. Unfortunately, it is messy to use in its crudest form, and
some people do not like it for this reason. Apart from the messiness,
though, it is an effective treatment, and some of the newer creams are
much more cosmetically acceptable. Scalp preparations, such as Polytar,
are useful and effective.

Steroid Creams

These preparations cause controversy among doctors and patients alike, because of their potential for side-effects. They are certainly effective in many cases of psoriasis, and some sufferers are so reliant on them that they will put a great deal of pressure upon their GP to continue to prescribe them.

In general, if a moderately strong steroid cream is used intermittently over a small area, it is unlikely to cause dangerous side-effects, such as thinning of the skin or suppression of the body's own steroid levels. Problems arise when the steroid creams are strong ones, cover a large area and are used over a considerable period of time. The skin may become permanently thin with multiple small 'thread veins' visible. Weight gain is another side-effect of large amounts of steroid being absorbed into the body, in the same way as if the steroid were taken as a tablet.

The other main danger of steroid creams is what happens when they are stopped. There can sometimes be a 'rebound' where the psoriasis, having been kept under control, bounces back and actually becomes worse than it was before. Caution is needed, therefore, when prescribing steroid creams and a need to use anything other than a small amount probably indicates that alternative treatment is necessary.

Dithranol (Trade Name: Dithrocream)

Dithranol has been in use for many years and has recently become more popular again. It has a potent effect on plaques, reducing their thickness by decreasing the rate of cell turnover. Like coal tar, it can irritate normal skin and needs to be applied carefully. It was originally used mostly as an overnight treatment, but is now prescribed for 'short contact' treatment where it is applied only for 20 to 30 minutes and then washed off. It is ideal for adults who have a small or moderate number of plaques, but is unsuitable for guttate psoriasis where there are many very small areas of affected skin.

Calcipotriol (Trade Name: Dovonex)

This is one of the newest treatments available on prescription from your GP. Its discovery came about during trials of treatments in patients with osteoporosis (thinning of the bones). A substance called alphacholecalciferol was administered to these patients to try and prevent bone thinning, and it was found that in those people who also had psoriasis, their skin improved. Calcipotriol cream was developed as a result. It is not entirely clear how it works, but it probably slows the rate of development of the keratinocytes, the cells at the top of the skin layer. It has recently been licensed for use in children, and can be used where the psoriasis covers up to 40 per cent of the body, that is mild to moderate disease. It can only be used for six weeks at a time, and a

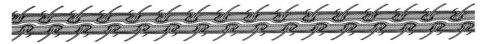

maximum amount per week is advised. Research on calcipotriol continues, but it is likely that it will become the main treatment for psoriasis in the future.

PUVA

For people with very widespread, resistant psoriasis, this treatment can be transforming in quite a short time. It is a very specialised treatment, and needs to be under the supervision of a dermatologist. A tablet treatment called psoralen is given, and a few hours later the patient is exposed to UVA which is a particular wavelength of ultraviolet light. The amount of exposure to UVA is increased gradually , according to response, to avoid burning. The two treatments combine to produce in the skin a substance which greatly reduces cell turnover. People who have this treatment generally feel very well afterwards. This is because it is very effective in just a few weeks and also because they get a suntan. One of the drawbacks, however, is the small increased risk of developing skin cancer in later life. This is still under evaluation, and many patients are followed up long term to assess the risk. However, for many severely affected psoriatics, it is undoubtedly a worthwhile treatment.

Tretinate, Methotrexate And Azathioprine

These are all drugs which are prescribed for severe psoriasis and need to be given under the close supervision of a dermatologist. They can all be used for other conditions, including arthritis and cancer, and their side-effects require careful monitoring. They are rarely prescribed in general practice.

Acne

Acne is probably the commonest skin complaint, and the one which causes the most upset among adolescents and young adults. A spotty skin can cause a good deal of psychological damage, and one study has even shown that it can affect youngsters' chances of finding employment. Like many skin conditions, it can range from the very mild, with just a few spots on the face, to very severe, requiring long-term specialist treatment.

Acne is caused by inflammation of the sebaceous glands, the glands in the skin which produce the fatty material to moisturise it (see figure 1 on page 16). It occurs mostly on the face, back and chest in young adults and adolescents, but a proportion of men and a few women need treatment into their thirties. About two-thirds of teenagers do not bother to see their GP for treatment, but buy skin creams or lotions over the counter. About 20 per cent, however, have spots which are bad enough to need medical advice and

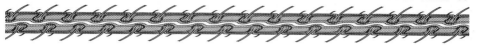

treatment.

A number of factors contribute to the formation of spots. First, production of the sex hormones *(androgens)* increases the size of the sebaceous glands and the amount of sebaceous material that is produced from the glands. This high rate of production of the fatty material *(sebum)*, causes the glands to become inflamed. A plug of cells blocks the exit to the glands and the contents of the glands may then be released deep in the skin causing even further inflammation. A particular bacterium, *Propionibacterium acnes*, is often present in skin with acne. This produces substances which also cause inflammation.

The acne may become so bad that nodules and cysts are formed, as well as scarring. About a fifth of sufferers have some degree of scarring.

While many teenagers improve once the initial surge of sex hormones is over at the end of puberty, it is possible to prevent quite a lot of scarring if treatment is appropriately given.

Treatment

Diet
It is a widely held belief that sweets and chocolate contribute to acne. However, it is the medical view, supported by some studies, that only rarely does chocolate cause the condition to worsen. It is common sense, however, to eat a balanced diet containing a variety of fresh fruits and vegetables to ensure that vitamins and minerals are in plentiful supply, enabling the body to fight infection and to heal the skin adequately. (see Chapter 3).

Topical Agents
Many of these can be bought over the counter in the form of antibacterial washes. Prescribable agents include Benoxyl Peroxide, which has some antibacterial action but also dries the skin. However, this can sometimes cause redness and irritation.

Topical Antibiotics
Topicycline, Dalacin T are two examples. Studies have shown them to be slightly more effective than peroxide, and they are suitable for use in mild to moderate acne, used once or twice daily. Some of these preparations are in roll-on form for convenience.

Antibiotics
Most people with more than mild acne will end up taking antibiotics. Over 80 per cent will respond to this treatment with a topical antibiotic

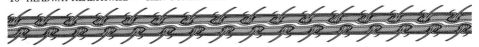

agent. The commonest antibiotic to be used is oxytetracycline, and similar drugs in this group are minocycline and doxycycline. A few people are allergic to tetracyclines, however, with rashes or other side-effects, and erythromycin or trimethoprim are both suitable antibiotics to use. In general, there is a 10 per cent improvement for every month of use and a course of six months' treatment, with review, is commonly recommended. Treatment starts with a fairly high dose and is then reduced to a maintenance dose. The more severe the acne, the higher the initial dose should be.

Hormone Therapy
For women, the drug cyproterone is available. Cyproterone acts on some of the sex hormones in the body (androgens) which increase the production of sebum. Cyproterone can cause damage to a developing foetus, however, and is therefore combined with oestradiol to give a contraceptive effect. The oestradiol also has a favourable effect on the sebaceous glands.

Studies have shown this therapy to be more effective than oxytetracycline, and it is a popular option for those women who require contraception anyway. However, like the oral contraceptive, it does not suit everybody, and may have the same side-effects that one expects with any contraceptive pill, including nausea and breast tenderness.

Isotretinoin
This treatment is reserved for very severe acne in which cysts and scarring are prominent. Because of its potentially severe side-effects, it is only prescribed by skin specialists, and the person taking this treatment needs to be monitored carefully. It acts by reducing the amount of sebum produced by the sebaceous glands by up to 90 per cent. It also reduces the bacterial count in the skin. Some of the side-effects include conjunctivitis (inflammation of the outermost front layer of the eye,) thinning of the hair and an increase in the level of blood fats.

Skin Cancers

Cancer of the skin has received a lot of recent media coverage. This is not surprising since the overall incidence of this cancer has doubled in the last twenty years. In sunny countries, such as Australia, it has reached almost epidemic proportions.

Most types of skin cancer, and particularly the more dangerous *malignant melanoma*, are related to exposure to the sun. We now know that burning of the skin, especially if it takes place in childhood, can greatly predispose an individual to skin cancer in later life. It is quite worrying, then, to hear of a recent survey by a

team of paediatric doctors in Sunderland who asked a number of mothers how often their children had been sunburnt in the previous year. While many had been sunburnt only once, nearly 10 per cent had suffered five times or more.

Unfortunately, it is still fashionable to have a tan in the UK, and many people are under the false impression that a tan provides protection against the sun's rays. A sustained campaign in Australia, by contrast, has considerably changed habits and attitudes over the last decade, and young adults, especially, are exposing themselves far less to the sun. The advice to 'slip on a tee shirt, slop on some sun cream and slap on a hat' is now going a long way to curb the high incidence of skin cancers in all age groups.

All of these skin cancers described below, if caught early, can be treated very successfully but, of course, prevention is a much better option. Using a sun cream whenever you are out in the sun, avoiding sunburn, especially in children, and keeping out of the sun between the hours of 11am and 3 pm should help to prevent skin cancer in later life.

Solar Keratosis

This is a condition that is precancerous, but the change to skin cancer is very slow and can take many years to happen. The area of skin becomes brown in colour and has a rough, irregular appearance. It usually occurs on skin previously exposed to a lot of sun, that is, the limbs or scalp.

Treatment with a cream called fluorouracil will usually get rid of the keratosis, but if there is any suspicion that it has changed to a tumour, it should be removed under local anaesthetic by a GP or specialist.

Bowen's Disease

Again, this condition is mostly linked to exposure to the sun and is precancerous. Although it occurs mostly on the limbs, it can affect any part of the body, including the breasts and abdomen. The areas of skin are usually brown and irregularly shaped. They look a bit like eczema. Anyone who has this condition should have a sample of the skin taken to check that there are no cancer cells present. It is then treated with fluorouracil cream or frozen with specially applied liquid nitrogen, which destroys the cells completely leaving normal skin to grow underneath.

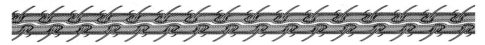

Malignant Melanoma

This is potentially the most serious of the skin cancers and, like the rest, is becoming more frequent. It can occur at any age, but is rare in childhood, becoming more common towards middle age. It arises from skin cells called melanocytes, which produces the pigment melanin, in skin.

Only a quarter of melanomas grow from moles already present on the skin. The rest occur on previously normal areas. Malignant melanomas usually arise in moles that are atypical in some way, that is, with an irregular edge or uneven pigment.

The danger signs to look for in a mole that may be turning into a melanoma are rapid changes in shape, colour or size. Over 90 per cent of melanomas show a change in all three. Other things to look for are crusting, bleeding or a change in sensation, usually a mild itching.

There are some risk factors which predispose towards this type of skin cancer. Anyone with a large number of moles and a family history of melanoma may have a greater risk, as well as those with a large amount of freckling. In women, a melanoma is more likely to appear on the legs. In men, it is more common on the trunk, and in the elderly on the face.

Treatment of a melanoma is by removing it and, depending on if it is small, this may be performed under just a local anaesthetic. If there is any doubt about the nature of the mole, it should be completely removed and sent off for microscopic examination. The thicker and larger the skin tumour, the more skin has to be taken off round it to be sure it has been got rid of. A skin graft may then be necessary if the area is large, and this would normally be done in hospital under a general anaesthetic.

Many people who are treated this way are completely cured. If there are any small, local recurrences they can often be dealt with by a laser rather than by further excision.

Basal Cell Carcinoma

This skin tumour is also known as a *rodent ulcer*, and is the most common skin malignancy. Like the other tumours, it is almost always the result of accumulative sun exposure. It occurs in older age groups as a rule, but may be seen from young adulthood onwards. A round, pearly-looking nodule usually appears on the face, particularly around the nose and eyes. It may have a raised edge and

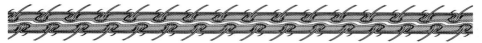

there may also be some crusting in the centre. For most people the best treatment is removal under a general anaesthetic by a plastic surgeon. It is important to remove these as they will continue growing rapidly if left untreated. Some tumours can be very successfully treated with radiotherapy, which is given to the very small area of the tumour and has few side-effects.

Squamous Cell Carcinoma

This is often found in people who work outdoors, and nearly always people who are over 55 years. It looks more crusty and opaque than a basal cell tumour. In its early stages, it may spread to other parts of the body, but this is rare. Otherwise, it is treated in a similar way to a basal cell tumour by surgical removal or by radiotherapy.

Benign Skin Conditions

Vitiligo

This condition affects approximately 1 per cent of the population worldwide and people with pigmented skin are more often affected. About a third of sufferers have a family member with the condition.

Patches of pale skin appear on various parts of the body, typically on the face, trunk and genital area. These patches are often symmetrically placed. They tend to enlarge slowly over a number of months or years, and only very rarely disappear again by themselves. Vitiligo, while itself quite harmless, is sometimes associated with general medical conditions, such as thyroid disease, diabetes, and Addison's disease, which is an underactivity of the adrenal glands. If you have the condition, it is worth seeking the advice of your GP to exclude these illnesses.

It is not known what causes this depigmentation of the skin, and research continues to look at the action of skin cells called melanocytes, which produce the pigment in our skin. For some reason, these cells stop functioning in the affected areas of skin. So far, very few treatments have had any effect.

Treatment

One treatment which has been used is PUVA (see page 38), and in a few people this has caused some repigmentation, but the overall results of the treatment have been disappointing.

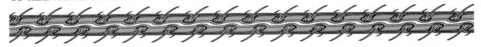

Many people with vitiligo are affected in the teenage years and girls, in particular, can find it very distressing, especially if it appears on the face. The most effective help is given by camouflage make-up, which conceals the pale patches totally when properly applied. Your doctor should know where to send you for this service which is provided on the NHS. Some creams and make-ups are available on prescription.

Seborrhoeic Warts

These benign growths occur on nearly everybody over the age of 40 years. They are round or oval, yellow, brown or black, and commonly occur on the trunk of the body. They tend to feel slightly greasy and may be attached to the skin by a stalk.

Treatment

As they never turn cancerous, they are only removed if they catch on clothing, or for cosmetic reasons. They can be frozen with liquid nitrogen or removed under a local anaesthetic.

Warts And Verrucas

These conditions are really one and the same, *verruca* being a term used for a wart on the sole of the foot. These are all caused by one of a number of viruses. They are common on the hands, face and feet and, although they look unsightly, are quite harmless. They cause a lot of anxiety among the parents of children who have them. It is sometimes difficult to accept that most warts disappear spontaneously in 12 to 18 months. They can cause discomfort in walking and some embarrassment if they are on the hands or face, so they are often treated.

Treatment

There are several liquid preparations, such as salicylic acid and gluteraldehyde, which need to be painted on regularly and then the wart is pared down either by the patient themselves or by the practice nurse or doctor. Cryotherapy is a rather quicker method, suitable for older children or adults. Liquid nitrogen is applied with a probe, which freezes the cells of the wart, thereafter forming a blister which finally drops off. Genital warts should be treated like any other sexually transmitted disease, and should be properly investigated by a specialist in infectious diseases. These are usually treated with 10 to 25% podophyllin in spirit, painted on then washed off after six hours.

NOURISH YOUR SKIN

You may not be able to judge a book by its cover, but your skin will reveal the state of your health. No matter how many layers of foundation, powder and cream, the tell-tale wrinkles and progressive lines on your face will give away your age.

Potions and lotions are all very well, but spare a thought for the most essential element in skin care – water. Just as a grape becomes a raisin as it dehydrates, so skin wrinkles if its moisture is lost. Try to drink at east eight glasses of water or other fluids per day to keep you hydrated and your skin healthy.

Protein intake is another requirement as, like all the other body tissue, the skin is made up of proteins. Indeed, a good mixed diet supplying all the essential nutrients, vitamins and minerals contributes greatly to all-round good health.

Foods rich in beta carotene and vitamin A help to regulate oil production and promote new cell formation – both essential for healthy skin. Vitamin A helps maintain soft skin and builds resistance to infections. A deficiency of beta carotene and vitamin A can result in flaky skin with clogged pores and spots, causes of many skin ailments. Vitamin C helps strengthen capillaries (delicate blood vessels) in the skin and promotes the healing of wounds. The B vitamins reduce facial oiliness and blackhead formation, and help to prevent eczema. Vitamin E improves the circulation in the facial capillaries, and generally aids in healing. Among the minerals, calcium gives soft, smooth skin, and iron improves pale skin. Potassium is good for dry skin, and zinc helps in healing.

Natural skin functions can be inhibited by the state of your overall health, and most ailments will affect the skin. For instance, stress can encourage a number of unsightly eruptions in the skin (at some stage), such as acne and rash. An underactive thyroid will give rise to rough, dry skin, and diabetics are prone to skin infections and eruptions. Then there are specific skin conditions, such as eczema and psoriasis, which are caused by imbalances in the body's systems.

The Free Radical Theory Of Ageing

One factor that cause wrinkles and ageing is free radicals. These are

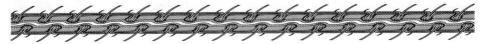

electronically unbalanced and highly reactive molecules that are responsible for weakening the immune system. There is considerable interest in the free radical theory of ageing, which was originated by Dr Denham Harman of Nebraska Medical Center. Free radicals attack the skin causing brown age spots and attack protein molecules causing *cross linking*, which is the main cause of wrinkles on the skin. Cross linking means that the free radicals create an abnormal chemical bond between protein molecules in the skin tissue.

How Free Radicals Are Created

Oxygen is necessary to sustain life but, paradoxically, it is also an agent that produces free radicals. All living things that use oxygen produce free radicals. Free radicals are the cause of rusting iron, hardened rubber and wrinkled skin. When cells use oxygen, they produce unstable molecules that lack an electron (molecules are stable only when they have an even number of electrons). These unstable oxygen molecules are free radicals. Created every minute we are alive, they are largely held in check by the body's own army of antioxidants, and as long as they are kept under control we remain healthy. However, if we begin to make more free radicals than we need (and they do serve a useful function in that they kill disease-causing bacteria), there is a risk of damage to the immune system and of developing chronic diseases.

Unchecked free radicals are thought to be the major cause of mutations and cancers, memory loss and senility, autoimmune diseases, ageing and wrinkles. The polyunsaturated fats that make up the body's cell walls are particularly sensitive to free radical attack. They become rancid (oxidised) and are structurally damaged.

Environmental Factors

As well as the body's normal production of free radicals, there are outside factors that can add to our free radical burden:

- excessive exposure to X-rays
- radioactive contamination
- pesticides, industrial solvents, CFCs and other pollutants

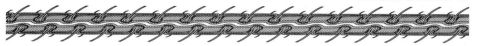

Neutralising Free Radicals

Free radicals can be hazardous to human health and, therefore, it is important to neutralise them before they do any damage. Protection from free radicals comes from *antioxidants*. An antioxidant is a substance that can protect foods – especially fats and oils – from oxidation (going rancid). It does this by preventing oxygen from combining with other substances and damaging cells.

The nutrients that are commonly thought of as our first line of defence against free radical attack are vitamins A, C and E, beta carotene, and the minerals zinc and selenium. (Some amino acids also have a part to play in fighting excess free radicals.) Vitamins (apart from vitamin D) and minerals cannot be produced by the body itself, and must come from the diet, so you can see how important is the relationship between sound nutrition and a healthy immune system.

The Body's Immunity

Through its immune system, the body has an amazing capacity to deal with the viruses, bacteria and other organisms that are around us every day of our lives. However, lack of nutrients can weaken the immune system and impair its function. To understand this is to understand the role of nutrition in the prevention of disease.

Our immune system is the body's main line of defence against both minor and major illnesses. As soon as the immune system encounters a germ or a bug that it perceives as foreign, certain cells in the body fight the organism to get rid of it. The system is so sophisticated that it can actually 'remember' the foreign organism and is able to respond to it more quickly the next time it is encountered. This is called *acquired immunity.*

Vaccination is a good example of one way we can acquire immunity. A small amount of treated or dead organism is introduced into the body by injecting a vaccine. As the organism is already treated or dead, there is no danger of acquiring the disease. However, as soon as the body's defence force encounters it, the immune system is put on red alert, fights it and makes antibodies to deal with it. The immune system will also remember how to get rid of the organism should it meet a similar one in the future. So, if you were to become infected with an active live organism of the same kind as the one used in the vaccine, say of cholera, your immune system will be able to respond to it before it has had a chance to

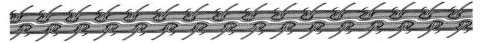

cause disease. All the information is stored in the thymus gland, the body's immune 'computer'. It instructs the body's defence force when to commence attack and, equally, when not to attack in the case of harmless foreign organisms.

As long as the immune system is healthy, it can fend off the onslaught of disease. But it can be compromised by poor diet, environmental pollution, stress and even the natural process of ageing, with serious consequences.

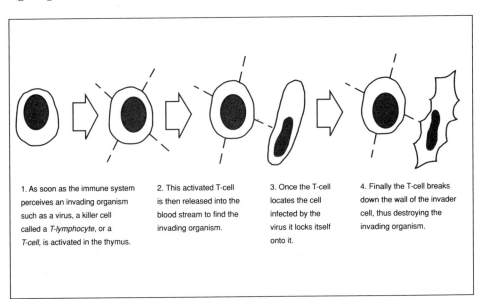

1. As soon as the immune system perceives an invading organism such as a virus, a killer cell called a *T-lymphocyte*, or a *T-cell*, is activated in the thymus.

2. This activated T-cell is then released into the blood stream to find the invading organism.

3. Once the T-cell locates the cell infected by the virus it locks itself onto it.

4. Finally the T-cell breaks down the wall of the invader cell, thus destroying the invading organism.

How the immune system works

Sometimes the system malfunctions, becomes overactive, and starts attacking harmless foreign substances. This is how allergy develops. Normally an allergen, such as pollen, is harmless and yet the immune system starts to attack pollen particles. The cells involved in allergic response come out in full force, releasing a substance called histamine, resulting in the symptoms of, for example, hay fever.

At times the immune system goes horribly wrong, and actually starts attacking the body's own cells. Rheumatoid arthritis is just such an example. Problems also arise in transplants because the immune system, programmed to reject foreign tissue, begins to attack the new heart or kidney.

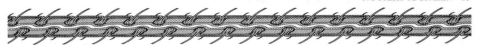

You can see how important it is to keep the immune system in a state of balance. However, the problem for the immune system in this late twentieth century is that while the human body is remarkably adaptable in its quest for survival, it needs time to change. Unfortunately, the pace of change in the environment has overtaken the body's natural ability to offer a timely response. The immune system is overworked and does not always know how to respond to the array of new enemies that confront it. Environmental pollution, the depletion of the ozone layer, pesticides and CFCs have all contributed in upsetting our finely-tuned immune system.

Furthermore, if the system cannot eliminate and neutralise a foreign organism or toxins, the body has to store it somewhere. The liver, bones, and even the brain, as well as the skin, can become the storehouses for this, sometimes dangerous, waste. The effects of these toxins, together with the imbalance of nutrients in our food, increases our vulnerability to disease.

Good Skin Care

Of the antioxidant nutrients, vitamin E is thought to be particularly beneficial in skin care. Pick up a 'natural' skin care preparation and you will find that vitamin E will often be included in the formulation. It is the moisturising properties of vitamin E which are best known. Applied directly to the skin in the form of creams, lotions and oils, it reduces water loss and maintains the skin's elasticity. It penetrates easily to the deeper skin layers, protecting nerve tissue, collagen, glands and blood vessels. Used in preparations in concentrations of up to 20 per cent, it is non-irritating and non-allergenic, even to the most sensitive skins.

Vitamin E is also found to be effective in healing the skin as well as keeping it looking good. Its anti-scarring properties have been used to treat burns, and dermatologists apply it to a variety of skin disorders. However, the most important role of vitamin E is as the protector of cell membranes. While we are alive, new cells are created and replace the cells which die. The younger we are, the more cells are created. As we reach our twenties, the number of new cells created is balanced by the number of cells that die. After that, as more cells die than are created, the ageing process sets in. Each cell is surrounded by a membrane that gives it shape as well as protection. The membrane also regulates the passage of materials in and out of the cells, and in this way is able to maintain a healthy

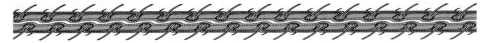

environment within itself. If the membrane is damaged, this delicate balance is disrupted and the cell may become diseased and may even die. As vitamin E helps to retain the integrity of this cell membrane, it is highly regarded as a skin protector.

Oil For The Skin

The older a skin becomes, the more oil it needs. The main function of oil is to trap in moisture and to prevent the skin from dehydrating. So it acts as a protector, and is essential for many aspects of skin health. There are several ways moisture can escape. The internal system may underfunction and fail to provide water to the skin or, as we age, the skin surface takes longer to replenish itself. The dry atmosphere created by central heating or very cold wind can all contribute to water loss. Coating our skins with oil can keep the moisture in and environmental hazards out.

For those whose oil-producing glands work overtime to produce oily skin, an external coating of oil actually helps, as it fools the glands into thinking that the skin has enough oil, thus regulating further production.

Application of oil to the skin can also be a way of feeding it with nutrients. Cold-pressed (heat extraction destroys vitamin E) wheatgerm oil, for example, has a high vitamin E content, as has the oil extracted from apricot kernels. Sesame and carrot oils contain pro-vitamin A. Evening primrose oil contains high levels of the fatty acid gamma linolenic acid (GLA), which helps to strengthen the structure of cell membranes.

Skin takes a lot of punishment and usually serves us well. A sound nutrition programme can go a long way in keeping disease at bay. However, the body can malfunction with resulting effects on the skin. Nutritional measures can help here, too. The rest of this chapter covers the common conditions and describes how they can be managed nutritionally.

Skin Infections

Boils, Abscesses, Cellulitis And Impetigo

All these conditions are most likely to appear when you feel run down, tired, weakened by poor diet or are suffering from diabetes or a blood disorder. They indicate a weakness in the immune system.

Recurrent attacks are symptomatic of a depressed immune system, which can be caused by nutritional deficiencies, allergies and excessive consumption of refined carbohydrates. Therefore, dietary measures to boost the immune system are of utmost importance. Substances that depress the immune system should be avoided. Zinc and vitamin A can be particularly helpful in the treatment of recurrent boils.

Supplements:
- vitamin C, 1 to3 g per day
- beta carotene, 15 to 30 mg per day
- zinc, 20 mg per day

Shingles And Cold Sores

Both are among the 70 viruses that compose the *herpes* family. As with bacterial infections, dietary factors which strengthen the immune system would undoubtedly help to manage these viral infections. Beta carotene is known to inhibit viruses, and to stimulate the white cells to combat viruses and increase the number of T-helper cells (which help other cells) in the immune system. Supplementation with vitamin C and zinc have also been shown to be effective in dealing with viral infections.

It has been found that foods rich in the non-essential amino acid *arginine* (one that can be made by the body and does not have to be obtained directly from food) increase the likelihood of a herpes lesion (wound) in those persons infected with the virus. Arginine-rich foods include peanuts, almonds, brazil nuts and cashews. A diet low in arginine has been adopted by many herpes sufferers to help control the infection. Conversely, an essential amino acid lysine (one that cannot be made by the body and must be obtained from the diet) has been found to be helpful in managing herpes infections. Vitamin C also offers protection.

The arginine/lysine theory of control is controversial, but nutritionists believe that such an approach could be effective. Studies have shown that the virus is dependent on adequate levels of arginine and low levels of lysine, so lysine supplementation and arginine avoidance seem appropriate. Experts believe that a fundamental factor in the success of low arginine and high lysine lies in the balance between the two, but finding this balance for each individual is a matter of trial and error. Foods that have a high lysine content are most fruit and vegetables (except peas), brewer's

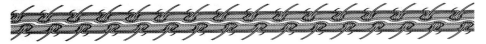

yeast, beans, cottage cheese, fish and other seafoods, as well as beef, lamb and poultry.

Eczema

While the primary cause of eczema is still unknown, dermatologists have long been aware of an association between diet and eczema. There is a number of studies that indicate that food allergy is an important predisposing factor. Other allergic disorders, such as asthma and hay fever, as well as emotional factors all have a part to play in the onset of eczema. Known culprits that may exacerbate eczema are cow's milk, eggs, wheat, fish and nuts. In many cases, exclusion of offending items from the diet will prevent eczema from flaring out of control. A diet diary may help identify suspect foods. However, comprehensive exclusion diets should only be carried out under professional supervision, especially in the case of children.

Most nutritionists agree that a wholefood diet eliminating junk foods, artificial colourings and refined sugars, is likely to be beneficial. Saturated fats found in red meat, dairy products, eggs, biscuits and pastries should be avoided. If it can be tolerated, oily fish (trout, salmon, herring, mackerel and sardines) should be included in the diet, as should vegetable oils. The emphasis should be on fresh foods, including fruit and vegetables, nuts and pulses.

Supplementation

One safe dietary supplement that may be employed in the management of eczema is evening primrose oil. In order to understand why this is so one needs to look at the role of a special group of nutrients called *essential fatty acids* (EFAs).

The Role Of Essential Fatty Acids

The body needs fats to perform various metabolic functions. Some of these fats cannot be made by the body, so their presence in the diet is of the utmost importance ('essential'). Modern eating habits, food processing and intensive animal rearing practices result in a diet severely lacking in these essential fats. Patients with eczema, in common with other atopic conditions, appear to be deficient in EFAs.

There are two families of EFAs: one found mainly in seed oils, such as sunflower, borage and evening primrose oil, and the other

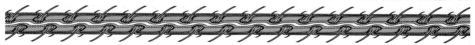

found mainly in fish oils.

The polyunsaturated fatty acids, such as linoleic acid (LA) and gamma linolenic acid (GLA), found in seed oils, and eicosapentaenoic acids (EPA), found in fish oils, have a very important role to play in the body. However, their production is inhibited by factors such as age, diet and hormonal conditions.

Diets high in saturated fats, cholesterol and trans fatty acids reduce the body's ability to produce these polyunsaturated fatty acids.

Two Major Functions Of EFAs

Converting Nutrients Into Energy

All cell membranes contain fats which are important for maintaining the integrity of the membranes. The fats also provide sites in which many physiological processes take place. If there is a deficiency of EFAs, the process in which nutrients are converted into body energy becomes inefficient. This lack of energy leads to poor growth and an impairment of body function.

Precursors Of Prostaglandins

Prostaglandins are hormone-like substances. It has now been established that they are produced from EFAs. They also help to regulate blood pressure, stimulate the immune system and maintain good cardiovascular function.

The Role Of EFAs In Disease Management

Dietary deficiency of EFAs results in altered membrane function, dermatosis, weight loss and eczema. Individual fatty acids have been used successfully in the management of a number of ailments. For example, supplementation with GLA has resulted in the successful treatment of eczema and other allergy-related disorders. Numerous studies are currently under way to evaluate the role of some of the individual polyunsaturated fatty acids in managing immune system-related disorders.

Evening primrose oil is an unassuming yellow flower that is known to possess remarkable health-giving properties because of the GLA content of its seeds. Most vegetable oils contain linoleic acid – an EFA. The normal diet is quite sufficient in it. However, before this EFA can be used by the body, it has to be converted via GLA to prostaglandin E1. Unfortunately, this conversion is fraught with

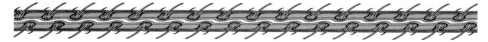

difficulties and can easily be blocked.

Viruses, cholesterol, saturated fatty acids, alcohol, insufficient insulin, radiation, vitamin and mineral deficiencies and the ageing process all contribute to blocking or adversely affecting this conversion.

As evening primrose oil has an unusually high amount of GLA, it can potentially avoid all these blockages. Such a source of dietary GLA can therefore be extremely valuable.

Further, if the body cannot make sufficient GLA and does not receive a dietary supply, then parts of the body system can be impaired. Evening primrose oil can help in conditions such as premenstrual syndrome (PMS), eczema and rheumatoid arthritis, and in controlling levels of cholesterol. The list is by no means exhaustive, and new research is now suggesting that ME (chronic fatigue syndrome) sufferers may also benefit, and so may hyperactive children and alcoholics.

Eczema is thought to be specifically associated with a deficiency of the enzyme needed to form GLA from linoleic acid, so a direct supply of GLA can be very useful. Research suggests that a minimum of four 500 mg capsules daily for adults and two a day for children is needed to relieve itching, but eight to twelve 500 mg capsules a day for adults and four a day for children is probably required to reduce the overall severity of the disease.

Hair, Skin And Nails

In a trial that examined the possibility of using evening primrose as a remedy for dry eyes, it was noted that the condition of skin, hair and nails often improved. Indeed, many people find evening primrose oil an internal beauty treatment, making skin softer, nails harder and hair stronger and shinier. And, in fact, evening primrose oil was found to help improve dry eyes.

Fish Oils

Fish oils have anti-inflammatory and anti-allergy effects. The importance of fish oils was discovered when two Danish scientists, John Dyerberg and Hans Bang, took samples of Eskimo blood during their journey to Greenland in 1976 when they accompanied Dr Hugh Sinclair, a nutritional biochemist who first discovered that Eskimos have very low blood cholesterol levels despite a diet which includes the highest animal fat content of any diet in the world.

When Dyerberg and Bang analysed the Eskimos' blood, they found that it contained high levels of the essential fatty acids *eicosapentaenoic* (EPA) and *docosapentaenoic acid* (DPA). These two, together with *docosahexaenoic acid* (DHA) are known as *omega 3 fatty acids*. Eczema, acne and psoriasis have all been found to have improved by the increase of fish oils in the diet.

Today we eat very little fish and, in particular, fatty fish such as mackerel and herrings, which are a primary dietary source of omega 3 essential fatty acids. Other similar sources are:

- sardines
- tuna (fresh)
- trout
- salmon

Nutritionists recommend that by decreasing our animal fat intake and increasing fish and vegetable oil consumption, we can achieve a considerable improvement in the incidence of eczema and related allergic and inflammatory disorders.

Vitamin A

Vitamin A is needed for the proper development and maintenance of the skin, and has a particular function in combating eczema. A deficiency of this vitamin results in hardening of the skin *(hyperkeratinisation)*, commonly found in eczema.

Zinc

Zinc is necessary for converting EFAs into anti-inflammatory prostaglandins and is, therefore, particularly important in the management of eczema. It is also involved in the production of skin cells and may, therefore, become deficient in cases of eczema because of the rapid cell turnover.

Vitamin C And Bioflavonoids

These are naturally occurring compounds in the skin or peel of citrus fruits and in some leafy vegetables. Among other things, these compounds control the release of histamine and other inflammatory agents, help to stabilise cell membranes, and decrease the contraction of smooth muscle. Consequently, they have been indicated for virtually all the allergic and inflammatory conditions.

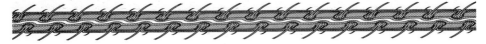

Vitamin C is instrumental in preventing the degeneration of collagen, the main protein in the connective tissue which makes up skin. As it is also a potent anti-oxidant and detoxifier, and so it is important in the management of eczema. In nature, vitamin C occurs in a 'package' with bioflavonoids, and each enhances the action of the other. A US study concluded that vitamin C in citrus extract was 35 per cent more available than vitamin C alone.

Supplementation For Eczema
- vitamin A, 7,500 iμ per day (pregnant woman should not take more than 2,500 iμ in supplement form)
- vitamin E, 400 iμ per day
- vitamin C with bioflavonoids, 500 mg of each per day
- zinc, 20 mg per day
- evening primrose oil, 2 to 3 g per day
- fish oils, 1 to 2 g per day

Urticaria (Hives) And Angio-oedema

This localised swelling of the skin is caused by the release of histamine within the skin. More than half of patients with hives develop a deeper and less-defined swelling called *angio-oedema*. This is a similar eruption to hives, but has large swollen areas which involve structures beneath the skin surface.

There are many different causes of urticaria and so its development cannot be ascribed to any one stimulus. Where there is a food allergy, there can be a number of factors that increase what passes through the gut wall – alcohol, aspirin, food flavourings and colourants and preservatives, for example.

Identifying and controlling all the factors that provoke an urticarial response is the basis of treatment and, where diet and nutrition are concerned, an elimination diet is the most useful approach. The diet should eliminate all suspected allergens as well as all food additives. Foods commonly associated with inducing urticaria are milk, eggs, fish, beans and nuts.

Food Colourants

One of the first food colourants to be reported as inducing urticaria was the azo dye, tartrazine. This is widely used in packaged foods as well as in a number of drugs, such as antibiotics and steroids.

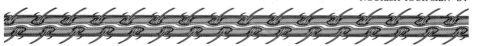

Food Flavourings

Salicylates are aspirin-like compounds that are used to flavour foods, such as ice-cream, chewing gum, soft drinks and cake mixes. Salicylates are also found in nuts and seeds and dried fruits such as raisins and prunes which have significantly high amounts. Herbs and spices, such as paprika, thyme, dill, oregano and turmeric, can also contribute to dietary salicylate.

Preservatives

Benzoates or benzoic acids are widely used as food preservatives, and are known to provoke reactions particularly in those who suffer from chronic urticaria. Shrimps and some fish have a high concentration of benzoates, which explains the incidence of adverse reactions to these foods.

Sulphites, used to keep processed foods from browning and to prevent microbial spoilage, have also been shown to induce urticaria. Sulphites are also sprayed on to fruits and vegetables.

Psoriasis

This condition, caused by the abnormal rate of division of cells, demonstrates the fact that the body's natural system is out of sorts. Incomplete protein digestion and impaired liver function are considered to be among the factors that contribute to this abnormal rate of cell division.

Protein Digestion

Incomplete protein digestion, or inadequate absorption of amino acids in the intestine, may lead to the proliferation of many toxic compounds as the bacteria in the large intestine try to break down the protein that has not been digested. Studies have shown that too many of the partial protein breakdown products known as *polyamines* can contribute to the excessive rate of cell division. In order to prevent the excessive formation of polyamines, it is necessary to ensure that protein digestion is complete. Dietary therapists may recommend supplementing with hydrochloric acids or pancreatic enzymes at mealtimes to aid protein digestion.

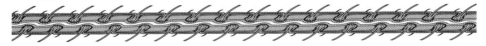

Impaired Liver Function

One of the liver's basic tasks is to filter blood. Herein lies the
connection between psoriasis and impaired liver function. Impaired
liver function means that there will be an increased level of toxins
circulating in the blood, and psoriasis is linked to excess toxicity.
Alcohol intake must be eliminated as it is known to worsen psoriasis
considerably. This is because it both increases the absorption of
toxins from the gut and impairs the function of the liver.

Dietary Considerations

Naturopaths (those who treat illness by stimulating natural healing)
seek to identify all the factors which contribute to psoriasis while
paying special attention to lifestyle and environmental factors. Some
practitioners may recommend a fast in which only water, herbal teas
and fruit and vegetable juices are allowed. Others advocate a
Schroth cure, based on a three-day cycle repeated over two or three
weeks. The dietary regime includes a high proportion of complex
carbohydrates (wholemeal toast or rolls, porridge, etc.) and no
fluids on the third day. These treatments would be followed by a
wholefood diet eliminating all processed foods and snacks
containing additives, high animal fat and sugar content, salt or
refined flour.

A Naturopaths' Recommended Psoriasis Diet

Breakfast
Compote of stewed apple, dates, blackberries and prunes.
Mixture of dates, apple and blackberries.
Porridge sweetened with molasses or honey and soya milk or prune
juice only.
Brown rice and/or barley (cooked) served with soya milk or stewed
apple.
Rye crispbread.

Lunch
Salad of any raw vegetables except tomatoes or peppers. Raw apple,
grated carrots, onions and garlic, cress and alfalfa seed sprouts are
especially good in salad.
1/4 to 1/2 lb of grated carrots every day for carotene.
Blended vegetable soup with Plantaforce as stock.
Two slices of rye crispbread or 1 slice of pumpernickel bread.
Jacket potato, brown rice and/or barley, millet, or millet and potato.

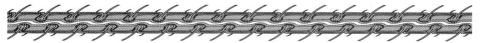

Dinner
Lamb – only once a week.
Beef – only once every 10-14 days.
Fish – once or twice a week
Take pulses and whole grains for protein requirement – including soya, haricot, aduki and kidney beans, lentils, chickpeas or tofu – in at least three meals per week.
At least two meals per week should consist of brown rice and vegetables and bean sprouts only.
Potatoes, brown rice, barley, millet or millet and potato.
Pumpkin.
Any fruit, except bananas and oranges.

Beverages
China or Earl Grey tea without milk or sugar.
Herb teas – drink one cup of sage tea per day. Elderflower tea is good, or try an infusion of elderflower, peppermint and a sprinkling of hops for flavour.
Drink 1 or 2 cups of fresh carrot juice per day.

Dressings, Oils And Condiments
Dress salads with Molkosan, olive oil, or cider vinegar.
Use garlic frequently in cooking and dressings.
Use only safflower, sunflower or olive oil, and then sparingly.
Use ample herbs, especially sage.
Use Herbamare salt.

Foods To Be Avoided
Chocolate, cheese, eggs, cows' milk, butter, yoghurt, processed foods, white flour, white sugar, cakes, biscuits, bread, citrus fruits, coffee, white flour products, red wine, excess alcohol, malt vinegar, smoked or pickled foods, yeast extracts, animal fats.
Smoking is prohibited.
   (Reprinted with kind permission of Naturopath Jan De Vries, from *Arthritis, Rheumatism and Psoriasis*, Mainstream Publishing.)

Supplementation

Zinc is found to be helpful because of its anti-inflammatory properties; a study has established that psoriatic patients have a low zinc/high copper ratio.

Essential Fatty Acids

Fish oils can be beneficial due to the high content of

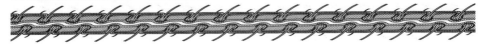

eicosapentaeonic acid. EPA is found significantly to improve psoriasis. In a study at the University of Aarhus in Denmark, 17 psoriatic patients were treated with *Super Gamma-Oil Marine* containing a combination of fish oils and evening primrose oil. After four months, excellent improvement was observed in 2 patients, moderate improvement in 8, mild improvement in 4, and no improvement in 3 patients. The skin of psoriasis sufferers contains a much higher level of inflammatory substances called *leukotrienes*. EPA helps to inhibit the production of these inflammatory compounds. Leukotrienes are derived from arachidonic acid which is found exclusively in animal fats, so it is very important to limit the intake of such fats.

Supplements
- vitamin A, 7,500 iμ per day
- vitamin D, 400 iμ per day
- vitamin E, 200 to 400 iμ per day
- selenium, 200 mcg per day
- zinc, 20 mg per day
- fish oil, 1 to 2 g per day *
- evening primrose oil, 2 to 3 g per day *
- * or use combined evening primrose oil/fish oil formula such as *Gamma Marine*

Acne

Natural therapists, unlike orthodox GPs, consider junk foods, such as burgers, chips and cola, not to mention sweets and chocolates, to be chiefly responsible for exacerbating acne in teenagers when hormone activity is at its peak. The impact of dietary habits has been vividly displayed in the difference between the incidence of acne in the Western world with its junk food culture as compared to cultures elsewhere in the world where junk foods are virtually unknown. Foods that are high in saturated fats, such as red meat, chocolate, etc., need to be replaced by fresh fruit and vegetables. Plenty of water before meals, yoghurt instead of ice-cream, are all sensible measures that can go a long way to alleviate the misery of acne.

Other causes of acne include a poor elimination of toxic substances through the bowels, impaired liver and kidney function, as well as poor expulsion of waste matter through the skin itself.

Bowel detoxification may be necessary to remove toxic bacteria

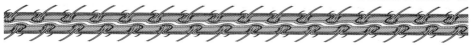

and to reseed *lactobacilli*, the friendly bacteria required by the body for digestion. Dietary fibre must also be increased to help speed food transit time and, therefore, avoid the build up of toxins in the body.

Nutritional Considerations

Eliminating all refined carbohydrates and reducing fat consumption is the starting point of any nutritional programme, as is the avoidance of foods containing transfatty acids – hardened margarines, shortening or oxidised fatty acids (re-used cooking oil).

Due to the combination of poor absorption and a poor diet, acne sufferers may be deficient in certain vitamins and minerals, such as vitamins A, B_6, E, zinc, chromium and selenium. A sensible supplementation regime of these nutrients can be helpful, particularly when they are not being obtained from food.

Vitamin A

Vitamin A has been shown to reduce sebum production, and a number of studies have demonstrated the effectiveness of this vitamin in treating acne. However, due to the high doses required, which can be potentially toxic, these should only be taken in consultation with a qualified professional. Another concern is the possibility of massive doses of vitamin A causing birth defects. Women of childbearing age need to take adequate birth control measures well before and after such treatment.

Vitamin B_6

Women with premenstrual aggravation of acne have been shown to be responsive to B_6 supplementation.

Vitamin E And Selenium

Males with acne have very low levels of the red blood cell enzyme, *glutathione peroxidase*. These levels can be normalised with supplementation of vitamin E and selenium. It is also thought that other antioxidants, for example, vitamin C and beta carotene, may also have a role to play in this process.

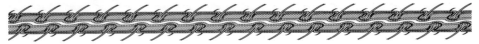

Chromium

According to dermatologists, insulin is thought to be effective in the treatment of acne. This suggests that acne may involve impaired glucose tolerance. Chromium works with insulin to metabolise sugar, and chromium-rich yeast has been shown to improve glucose tolerance and to enhance insulin sensitivity, and has been reported to improve the condition of acne sufferers.

Zinc

While there has been much controversy following a number of double-blind studies on the role of zinc supplementation in the treatment of acne, the importance of this mineral for normal skin function is well recognised, due to its involvement in inflammation control, hormone activation and immune system activity. Low zinc levels increase the conversion of the male hormone testosterone into a more potent form *(dihydroestosterone)*, which promotes acne. High levels of zinc inhibit this conversion.

Supplements

- vitamin A, 7,500 iµ per day (pregnant woman should not take more than 2,500 iµ in supplement form)
- vitamin B complex, 50 mg per day
- vitamin E, 200 to 400 iµ per day
- vitamin C, 1 g per day
- chromium, 200 to 400 mcg per day
- selenium, 100 to 200 mcg per day
- zinc, 15 to 20 mg per day

Skin Cancers

The increase in the incidence of skin cancers has primarily been attributed to excessive exposure to sunlight. The issue has become of even greater concern as the progressive depletion of the ozone layer has increased the levels of ultraviolet light to which the human body is exposed. However, experts now point to a number of dietary and environmental factors which contribute to the problem.

Evidence is accumulating that vitamin D inhibits melanoma and other skin cancers. The use of unnatural fat sources, such as margarine, may also affect the balance of the mechanisms which

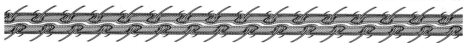

regulate the optimum fat composition of the skin. So the sorts of fat we consume may be an important factor in determining the incidence of melanoma.

There is evidence, too, that a deficiency of vitamin B_6 increases sensitivity to ultraviolet light. Vitamin B_6 levels in grains are considerably reduced in the milling and refining processes. (White bread contains only 22 per cent of the vitamin B_6 content of wholemeal bread.)

Dietary Considerations For The Prevention Of Cancer

While it is not within the scope of this book to discuss specific alternative treatments for cancers, dietary guidelines for its prevention are appropriate. One can do no better than to quote the recommendations of the American Cancer Society (ACS):

- Avoid obesity. Obese people run an increased risk of cancers of the uterus, stomach, kidney, gallbladder, colon and breast. A study by the ACS demonstrated that a man who is 40 per cent overweight has a 33 per cent greater risk of developing cancer compared to a man who is of normal weight. A woman who is 40 per cent overweight has a 55 per cent greater risk than a woman who is not overweight.
- Eat more high-fibre foods. High-fibre foods are generally rich in nutrients and low in calories and fat. Eating a variety of foods, such as fresh fruit, vegetables and whole grains, will provide the best source of vitamins and minerals as well as fibrous substances.
- Cut down on fat intake. Both saturated and unsaturated fats in excess have been found to promote cancer. Cutting back on fatty foods, fats and oils also helps to maintain correct body weight as they are the major sources of superfluous calories.
- Cut down on alcohol. In addition to causing liver cancer, alcohol abuse also increases the risk of cancers of the mouth, larynx and oesophagus. This risk is even greater in alcohol abusers who smoke. It also dilates blood vessels, increasing sensitivity to sunlight.
- Reduce consumption of smoked and salt-cured and nitrite-cured foods. Nitrates and nitrites are common preservatives used in meats. They are also used to cure or pickle foods. These chemicals can form *nitrosamines* which, in turn, cause cancer.
- Increase intake of foods rich in beta carotene and vitamin C in the daily diet. Carrots, spinach, apricots, peaches and tomatoes are all rich in beta carotene, a precursor of active vitamin A, which has been shown to decrease the risk of cancers of the larynx, oesophagus and lung.

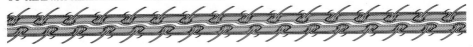

A diet that contains adequate amounts of foods rich in beta carotene, such as dark green leafy vegetables, carrots and apricots, has been found to reduce the risk of cancer. Dark green or orange vegetables and fruits contain beta carotene. This plant pigment is converted into vitamin A in the body.

Vitamin C is another anti-cancer vitamin. Those who consume vitamin C-rich foods, such as citrus fruits, have a reduced risk of stomach and throat cancers. Vitamin C also inactivates the cancer-causing nitrosamines. Found in cigarettes, smoked meat and processed foods, the nitrates are converted into nitrosamines in the absence of vitamin C. The presence of vitamin C blocks their formation, thus reducing the risk of developing cancer.

Finding A Practitioner Who Can Help With Dietary Recommendations

The British Naturopathic and Osteopathic Association, 6 Netherall Gardens, London, NW3 5 RR, maintains a register of qualified practitioners who have followed a four-year course at the British College of Naturopathy and Osteopathy.

The British Society for Nutritional Medicine, 4 Museum Street, York, YO1 2ES, maintains a register of qualified medical professionals as well as associate members who are qualified members of the related professions.

The Nutrition Association, 36 Wycombe Road, Marlow, Buckinghamshire, SL7 3HX, maintains a register of practitioners of nutrition and diet therapy. Or consult:

The Nutrition Consultants Association, c/o The Institute of Optimum Nutrition, 5 Jerdan Street, London, SW6 1BE or

The Society for the Promotion of Nutritional Therapy, First Floor, The Enterprise Centre, Station Parade, Eastbourne, BN1 1BE.

Further Reading

Naturopathic Medicine by Roger Newman Turner (Thorsons)
Viruses, Allergies and the Immune System by Jan De Vries (Mainstream Publishing)
Arthritis Rheumatism and Psoriasis by Jan De Vries (Mainstream Publishing)
Vitamin Guide by Hasnain Walji (Element Books)
E for Additives by Maurice Hanssen (Thorsons)

Home Skin Care Programme

Your kitchen can offer many possibilities for natural skin care.

Avocado

Rich in mono-unsaturated oils, avocados make a healthy addition to the diet from the outside as well as the inside. To make a rich after shampoo conditioner, mash together one ripe avocado, some honey and a little avocado or olive oil. Spread thickly on the hair and rinse off after 5 or 10 minutes.

Cucumber

Use slices of cucumber to pep up tired eyes. Or grate a quarter of a cucumber, squeeze it to extract the juice and mix it with a cupful of milk. Use the mixture with cotton wool as a cleanser – ideal for normal to oily skin. Cucumber juice also makes a cooling addition to your basic skin cream.

Milk

Soothe away tension in a warm, moisturising bath with added milk – perhaps not as many tons of asses' milk as Cleopatra used, but a cup or two of silver top will do just as well.

Oats

A staple food of the Scots and recently in vogue for its high content of soluble fibres, which may have cholesterol-lowering effects, oats can also be made into a useful body scrub. Make a gentle scrub by mixing oats with honey, yoghurt and ground almonds into a paste – good enough to eat!

Water

Drink as much pure, fresh water as you can. It will cleanse your skin from the inside out. Or spray a fine mist of water over your face before moisturising to seal in the moisture and retain a youthful look.

Yoghurt

Egyptian women have used it for thousands of years as a cleanser and beauty aid. Live yoghurt contains bacteria which in turn kill the bacteria that may contribute to spots and blemishes. Apply natural yoghurt to the face and skin, relax and leave it on for 5 to 10 minutes before rinsing it off and moisturising.

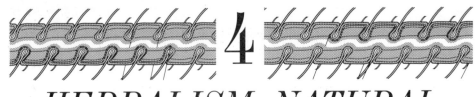

HERBALISM: NATURAL SKIN CARE

Long before the advent of modern synthetic drugs, healing with herbs was a widespread and highly-regarded practice. Chinese and Egyptian records going back almost 5,000 years show that plants were 'catalogued' according to the specific diseases for which they could be used. In China and India today, herbalism remains in the mainstream of healing practice. But the type of herbalism practised in those countries reflects the belief that the human being must be viewed as a whole. This gives rise to the concept that the attributes of the herbs to be used must match the attributes of the disease.

In the Western world, the use of herbs was common, too, and herb gardens flourished in monasteries in medieval times. The advent of the printing press brought in its wake a plethora of compilations and publications of herbals and, right up until the nineteenth century, herbal medicine was the most commonly used method of healing. The National Association of Medical Herbalists was founded in 1864 (now the National Institute of Medical Herbalists); at this time almost all medicines were plant-based. Only since the 1940s have synthetic drugs superseded plant-based medicines.

It is beyond the scope of this book to discuss the issues in the modern context but, among others, the National Institute of Medical Herbalists and the Natural Medicines Society (the consumer organisation), have been involved in negotiations and continue to play an active part in ensuring that the right of the consumer to choose which system of medicine he or she prefers is not taken away.

Many of the twentieth-century synthesised drugs have their origins in plant materials, so it must be acknowledged that modern medicine has its roots in herbal medicine. Plants are still used as a source of active ingredients which are then analysed, synthesised and used as potent drugs. For example, aspirin was discovered in the last century in plants such as meadowsweet and willow, and steroids are synthesised from a chemical extracted from the wild yam.

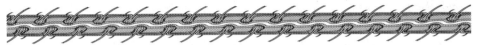

Medical Herbalism – A Holistic Approach

In common with other complementary therapies, herbal medicine offers a holistic approach in which you are treated not only for the symptom, but also for the cause of the symptom.

Furthermore, herbalists consider that isolating a substance from its surrounding properties, as with the synthetic versions in modern drugs, renders the substance more potent and, therefore, more dangerous. Herbal practitioners believe that natural remedies run less risk of producing side-effects. Not only are herbal compounds less potent, but they also contain other substances created naturally within the herb that can neutralise the potential danger of the active ingredient in the plant. Herbalists do not claim that all herbal medicines are entirely safe, as many are known to be toxic if taken in high doses, but they are generally reckoned to be far safer than orthodox medicines by herbalists.

The diagnostic techniques of many medical herbalists resemble those of GPs, using the same methods and equipment. But as well as considering the presenting symptoms, the herbalist also attempts to evaluate the overall balance of the body's systems. When presented with a set of symptoms, a herbalist is concerned to discover what the body is trying to do for itself when it manifests those symptoms. For example, eczema is, on one level, seen as a good sign. It means that the patient's constitution is strong because the disharmony in the body is being expressed by the most superficial organ of the body. It indicates that the imbalance has not gone inwards where it can have more serious consequences. A herbalist will look deeper and consider the state of the immune system, and will prescribe herbs that assist the body in what it is trying to do and which support the immune system. A very apt description of the herbalist's view of an infection as compared to that of a GP is offered by Dr Stephen Fulder in *The Handbook of Complementary Medicine.* He writes:

> For example, an infection may point in the first place to "stagnation" of the affected tissues. Healthy tissues, like running water, cannot suffer colonisation by bacteria; such an invasion can only occur in the histological equivalent of a brackish pond. Treatment of infections then demands that the tissue be "cleansed" and brought back into vital circulation. Antibiotics would only be necessary in this scheme if the colonisation was so excessive that there was real doubt as to the host's ability to overcome it from vital resources, and then appropriate only if the underlying stagnation were treated as well. Using antibiotics alone is seen as being as productive as pouring disinfectant into the brackish

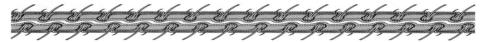

pond and declaring it 'clean'.

(Fulder, S, *Handbook of Complementary Medicine*, Oxford University Press, 1988, p. 178)
by permission of Oxford University Press

Just as symptoms vary from person to person, so must herbs be chosen according to the person's disposition and symptoms. Each herb has its own therapeutic property and medical herbalists have centuries of experience to fall back on in identifying these properties. Herbal medicine aims not merely to relieve the symptoms of disease, but also to approach the root cause of the problem itself, often by creating the conditions that mobilise the body to exercise its own capacity for healing.

The therapy considers not only the physical but also the mental and spiritual aspects of treatment, and so a medical herbalist would consider it important to have regard to the social and economic conditions that might perpetuate ill health in the person.

The skill of the practitioner lies in recognising that what may work for one person may not necessarily work for another. So entirely different remedies may successfully be given to treat two patients apparently suffering from the same complaint. Many herbalists are reporting an increase in the incidence of allergic conditions, and this is viewed as a consequence of our immune systems being severely compromised by a diet rich in refined foods and sugar, and deficient in vitamins, minerals and essential fatty acids. Consequently, herbalists also give advice on diet and supplementation in addition to the herbal prescription.

What Is A Herb?

Most of us think of herbs as being the plants used in cooking to add flavour to food, but to a botanist a herb is a non-woody plant that is under 30 cm high while, to the gardener, herbs are ornamental plants used as decoration in a herbaceous border. However, to a medical herbalist, a herb is any plant material that can be used in medicine and health care. So not only are botanical herbs used in herbal medicine, but also all the anatomical parts of plants, including seeds, the bark of a tree and the flowers. Even ferns, mosses, fungi and seaweed are classified as herbs.

Western herbal remedies usually use a single herb for a specific condition, although herbal compounds are sometimes administered. Other systems, especially the Chinese, make greater use of herbal prescriptions in carefully formulated combinations. Of

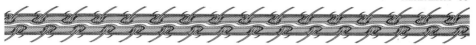

course, there are also the 'fast food' herbs available in tablet form from health food shops.

Herbal preparations are not only ingested orally as pills. Herbal tisanes and teas prepared by infusing the herbs are alternative methods of administration, as are herbal baths. Herbal medication can be taken in the form of syrups or extraction drops to be held under the tongue where they can be absorbed quickly through the mucous tissues. Herbs can also be inhaled through steam inhalation.

How Does Herbal Medicine Work?

As with the other symptoms of alternative health care, explaining exactly how herbal medicine works is difficult. Some things work and yet there is no scientific proof as to why they work. Herbs are believed to maintain good health by stimulating the body's own powers of healing, and to promote good health by toning the organs and nourishing the tissues and blood.

Herbs And The Skin

The skin acts to protect the body from infections by secreting antimicrobial secretions and by harbouring friendly bacteria. It is responsible for maintaining a harmonious inner environment by preventing the loss of water, salts and organic substances from inside the body, while acting as an excretory route for the expulsion of waste products and excess water. The skin's functions are complex and intricately tied up with other bodily organs, so disorders can be connected with malfunctions in other parts of the body.

Because skin problems reflect a variety of both internal and external conditions, there are many different herbs available for treatment. It is possible, however, to mark out particular groups of herbs which are helpful for skin problems.

Modern herbal practice, though more sophisticated than its Victorian counterpart, still uses the Victorian classifications which are based on the plants' physiological processes. *Vulneraries* promote the healing of fresh cuts and wounds, and have astringent qualities which arrest bleeding and condense tissue. *Alteratives* work gradually as 'blood purifiers', improving nutrition and restoring a healthy functioning in the body, while *antimicrobials* help the body to destroy or resist pathogenic micro-organisms that

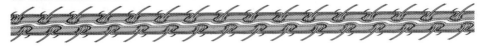

have invaded or which act on the skin. *Diaphoretics* promote perspiration and *diuretics* increase the secretion and expulsion of urine. Both of these aid the excretory process. *Nervines* soothe the nerves, and are also commonly used for skin complaints. *Hepatics* act on the liver.

Eczema

Whether the eczema is contact eczema, also known as dermatitis, a local allergy reaction, or atopic eczema, herbs can help to alleviate symptoms, although a holistic approach needs to be adopted to cure the root of the problem. This is particularly so when dealing with allergies. The allergen has to be identified and removed for the herbal support to be effective, so changes in diet and lifestyle may be an integral part of the treatment.

Herbal remedies are selected according to individual needs, but traditionally, herbs such as burdock root, figwort, fumitory, mountain grape, nettle, pansy and red clover, taken internally, have a good reputation for the treatment of eczema. Many of them are alteratives for cleansing and purifying bodily functions. A suggestion for a good internal remedy is to make a basic mixture of figwort, nettle and red clover, to be drunk as a tea three times daily. Marigold is similarly reckoned to be useful in treating eczema. An infusion can be made by adding 30 g of marigold flowers to a pint of boiling water. Strain and drink. It is said to relieve itching, blistering and flaky skin. The application of marigold or chickweed ointment, available from chemists and health food shops, can also alleviate such symptoms.

External treatments for eczema in the form of ointments and compresses may contain herbs such as burdock, chickweed, comfrey, golden seal, pansy, witch hazel and marigold. Burdock makes a good basic ointment. Simply compress the sap of a fresh root and mix with petroleum jelly to the right consistency. Apply to the affected areas.

Psoriasis

The cause of psoriasis is difficult to fathom, and can be due to physical or psychological factors. Lifestyle and stress levels also need to be taken into consideration when diagnosing and reviewing treatment. Most of the herbs recommended for psoriasis

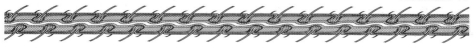

are alteratives, and these include burdock root, cleavers, mountain grape, red clover and sarsaparilla, while hepatics, such as dandelion and yellow dock, and diuretics, such as cleavers or figwort, may also be used. Nervines are helpful in conditions where it is necessary to strengthen the nerve response to stress, and herbs such as motherwort, lime flowers, mistletoe, skullcap and valerian, are available. Combinations of these herbs may be made up by the practitioner, depending on individual circumstances. For relief of the symptoms, ointments made from comfrey, chickweed or marshmallow are beneficial.

Acne

The underlying causes of acne are generally hormonal or dietary, and treatment is prescribed in the light of this. The herbal approach aims to balance food metabolism and to help the body rid itself of the wastes which may be causing the condition. Alteratives, such as figwort, cleavers, red clover, mountain grape and yellow dock, are beneficial, as are antimicrobials, such as echinacea, and hepatics, such as blue flag and dandelion. A suggested mixture consists of taking, in equal parts, blue flag, cleavers, echinacea and figwort as a tea to be drunk three times daily.

Herbs can also be used in the making of anti-inflammatory and anti bacterial skin washes. *Infusions* (a tea that you brew and drink) or *tinctures* (made by crushing and steeping a herb in alcohol for about ten days, after which the liquid is strained) of calendula, chamomile or a mixture of yarrow, elder or lavender dabbed on to the skin may help. Herbal steam baths may also help to clear affected areas. Chamomile, lavender, lime flowers or sage flowers are amenable to this purpose.

Urticaria Or Hives

A cool infusion of chickweed or chamomile may help to relieve itching, while herbs such as yarrow, golden seal, gentian and chamomile, are recommended for improving the functioning of the liver and digestive system.

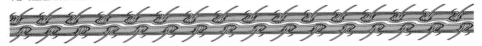

Bacterial Infections

Boils

Boils may be treated by using herbs both externally and internally, as it is vital to enhance the body's innate vitality and resistance as well as helping the body to get rid of bacteria. Usually, a combination of antimicrobials and alteratives is used. Specifically, echinacea, pasque flower and wild indigo are traditionally used for the treatment of boils, and are used in combination to aid the lymphatic system. An infusion of two parts echinacea, two parts wild indigo, and one part pasque flower, to be drunk three times daily, is a typical remedy. For self-help, an ointment or poultice can be made to draw pus from the boil. Marshmallow leaf or cabbage leaf, with echinacea or myrrh to control the infection, are effective herbs to use.

Impetigo

Impetigo is dealt with through the use of antimicrobials, supported by alteratives and tonics, with external applications of a lotion of echinacea, marigold, myrrh and wild indigo, which can be used to combat the infection and help to rebuild ecological barriers. Scrupulous hygiene and a wholesome diet are essential.

Styes

Styes may be treated by making a *decoction* (the roots, seeds, stems and other parts of the plants that are boiled in water) of eyebright and chamomile, to help reduce the inflammation. Marigold can be taken internally to stimulate the lymphatic system.

Viral Infections

Cold Sores

Cold sores can be tackled with a good diet, high vitamin C supplementation and through supporting the body's eliminative processes. A herbal mixture, such as two parts cleavers, two parts echinacea and one part oats, to be drunk as a tea twice daily, will assist.

Warts

Warts can be treated with a herbal remedy consisting of lymphatic cleansers and tonics. The traditional herbs for the treatment of warts are cleavers, garlic, prickly ash or wormwood. External treatment for the quick removal of warts involves the herbs dandelion, used by expressing the white juice from fresh stems and applying directly, and thuja, made into a tincture or lotion and then applied.

Fungal Infections

Athlete's Foot

Athlete's foot may be treated with daily herbal footbaths. Infusions of golden seal root or a combination of red clover, sage, calendula and agrimony with two teaspoons of cider vinegar can help. Calendula lotion applied to the affected area or direct application of tea tree or eucalyptus oil is also beneficial.

Ringworm

Ringworm can be treated internally with a herbal mixture that raises the body's resistance and increases lymphatic drainage. One suggestion is a mixture of two parts echinacea and one part each of cleavers, wild indigo and yellow dock, in a tea to be drunk three times daily. Externally, anti fungal herbs can be applied directly. These include eucalyptus, garlic, golden seal, marigold, myrrh and thuja.

Finding A Practitioner

The Professional Medical Herbalist

Practitioners are usually members of the National Institute of Medical Herbalists and apply Western herbal medicine in a consulting room. The diagnostic techniques of many qualified medical herbalists resemble those of GPs, using the same methods and equipment for blood pressure, pulse taking, physical examination and assessment of urine and blood samples.

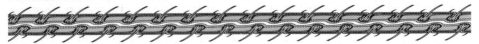

The National Institute of Medical Herbalists, 9 Palace Gate, Exeter, EX1 1JA.
The General Council and Register of Consultant Herbalists, Marlborough House, Swanpool, Falmouth, Cornwall, TR11 4HW.

Chinese Herbalists

Traditional Chinese herbalists tend to be confined to Chinese centres, practising mainly within the Chinese community. There is also the 'modern' practitioner of Chinese herbalism who uses herbs in conjunction with acupuncture.
Register of Chinese Herbal Medicine, 138 Prestbury Road, Cheltenham, GLS2 2DP.

Ayurvedic And Unani Practitioners

Commonly known as *Vaids* and *Hakims*, these practitioners are mainly found within the Indian and Pakistani communities, and offer treatment based on traditional principles.

Further Reading

A–Z of Modern Herbalism by Simon Mills (Thorsons)
Herbalism: Headway Lifeguides by Frances Büning and Paul Hambly (Hodder & Stoughton)
Herbal Medicine by Dian Dincin Buchman (Rider Books)
Potter's New Cyclopaedia of Botanical Drugs by R C Wren (C W Daniel)
The New Holistic Herbal by David Hoffman (Element Books)
Thorson's Guide to Medical Herbalism by David Hoffman (Thorsons)
Traditional Home Herbal Remedies by Jan de Vries (Mainstream Publishing)

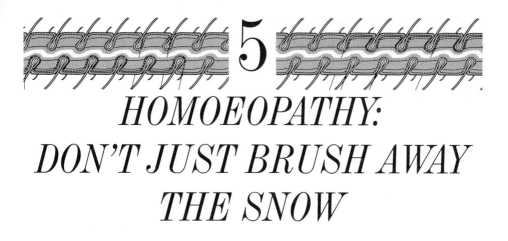

HOMOEOPATHY:
DON'T JUST BRUSH AWAY
THE SNOW

'Like cures like.' This is the essence of homoeopathic medicine, which adopts a holistic approach in not only alleviating symptoms, but also dealing with the causes of illness and health regeneration. The ultimate aim of homoeopathic treatment is to enable a person to reach a level of health where there is no longer any dependence on medicine or therapy.

Homoeopathy has its roots in ancient times. The writings of the Greek physician, Hippocrates, reflect certain homoeopathic principles while Paracelsus, a sixteenth-century philosopher and physician, said that, 'Those who merely study and treat the effects of disease are like those who imagine that they can drive away winter by brushing snow from the door. It is not the snow that causes the winter but the winter that causes the snow.' He was, in fact, espousing a vital tenet of homoeopathy, that symptoms are not actually manifestations of a disease, but the effects of the body's attempt to cure itself.

Homoeopathy was developed in the late eighteenth century by the German doctor, Samuel Hahnemann, who stopped practising orthodox medicine which he considered to be brutal, pointless and, more significantly, often fatal. In his day, the practice of bleeding patients, administering strong enemas and the use of poisonous drugs were common, and resulted in a high patient death rate. He was drawn towards homoeopathic principles after reading about the role of quinine *(cinchona)* in the treatment of malaria. His curiosity aroused, Hahnemann dosed himself liberally with quinine for several days and developed the symptoms of malaria, thus establishing that not only could quinine treat malaria, but that also large doses of quinine could cause malarial symptoms in a healthy person.

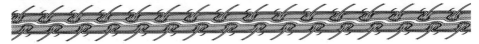

Over a period of time, Hahnemann went on to experiment with other drugs, trying them on himself and on his family. He called these experiments *provings* and noted each individual person's reaction to the drugs. His research led him to criticise orthodox medicine heavily and, in particular, the treatment of an illness with its opposite. He argued that the remedy for the healing of a disease should be one that artificially produces a disease as similar as possible to the first one. From this comes the philosophy of *similia similibus*, like with like, in medical practice.

Homoeopathy grew, though not without considerable opposition from the orthodox medical profession. However, its value was highlighted during the various cholera epidemics in Europe when Hahnemann treated, with great success, cholera victims with a homoeopathic solution of camphor. By the time of Hahnemann's death in 1843, homoeopathy had spread over most of continental Europe and had reached Russia, South America, Britain and parts of the USA.

How Homoeopathy Works

There is a fundamental difference between homoeopathic and allopathic (conventional) medicine in the way symptoms are viewed. Homoeopaths regard symptoms as an adaptive response by the body in defending itself and as a sign of the disease, while allopathic practitioners see the symptom as the disease. Since homoeopathy looks at the symptom as the way in which the body expresses its reaction to the underlying disorder, the homoeopath's task is to prescribe a remedy that will stimulate the body to heal itself more quickly. The correct remedy is one that will create similar symptoms in a healthy person when given in material doses. Homoeopathy is based on the following three principles.

The Law Of Similars

The mental, emotional and physical aspects of a patient's condition are analysed as part of a unified effort to resolve an inner disturbance and to return to a state of balance. The homoeopath prescribes a remedy which, through previous testing on healthy people and from clinical experience, is known to produce a similar symptom picture to that of the patient. This

prescribed similar remedy then stimulates and assists the patient's own natural healing efforts.

The Single Remedies

Although symptoms appear to be localised, homoeopaths believe that it is the patient's whole system which is out of balance and is striving to return to health, and that this whole can only be stimulated by a single remedy at any one time. The single remedy allows the homoeopath to observe clearly and to evaluate its effect before a further prescription is considered.

The Minimal Dose

Due to the similarity between the remedy's known symptom picture and that of the patient's, the patient is highly sensitive to its stimulus and so only a minute dose is needed in the form of a 'specially prepared potency'. The potency and the number of doses is determined by the homoeopath according to the needs of the individual patient.

The greatest debate and controversy surrounding homoeopathy is the concept of dilution. Homoeopathic remedies are diluted to such a degree that it is inconceivable that any of the original substance is left at all. Sceptics therefore question how such a remedy can work. Many homoeopaths readily admit that they do not know how it works, but merely that it does. As Hahnemann stated, 'Homoeopathy is not founded on theory; it is purely and simply a therapeutic rule based on observed facts.'

Some say that looking for a physical explanation ignores the holistic nature of the therapy, and that it may well be the case that these high potencies may be acting at a subtle level of energy like the *chi* in Chinese medicine or the *prana* in Ayurvedic medicine. It is argued that the remedies resonate with a person's 'vital force', like the *chi* or the *prana*. A healthy person vibrates at a certain energy frequency, which is more harmonious than that of an unhealthy person. The right homoeopathic remedy is like a boost of subtle energy, which returns the body to its proper energy frequency and so helps an ill person. When a body is in tune, resonating at its proper rate, it is able to use its immune system to throw off the toxins that cause illness.

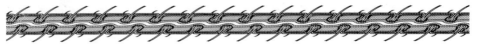

How Homoeopathic Remedies Are Made

Homoeopathic remedies can be prepared from anything that causes the desired symptoms. Indeed, a prescription for a cold with a runny nose and a bad throat could be *Allium cepa,* a homoeopathic preparation made from red onion. Why it is effective is clear when we consider what happens when we cut up an onion. We experience a runny nose, stinging in the throat and in the eyes, symptoms similar to those of a cold.

Most homoeopathic medicines are derived from plants, but minerals are also used.

After preparation of the raw materials, the remedies are made by serial dilution and *succussion* (vigorous shaking). Each stage of succussion increases the potency, which is given a number and a letter. Potencies with a 'X' affix are diluted 1:9, and those with a 'C' affix are diluted 1:99 at each successive stage. Once the substance becomes soluble in a strong dilutant, it can be used from then on.

How The Remedies Are Given

Remedies tend to be prescribed according to which strength or potency is required. (The lower potencies have been subjected to less dilution than the higher ones.) There is a growing number of outlets for the sale of homoeopathic medicines, and many high street chemists now stock basic homoeopathic medicines, as do many health food shops. Remedies are available in the form of tablets, granules, pilules, powders or in liquid form, while creams and ointments are available for external use. Generally, the homoeopathic medicines that are available over the counter are low potencies, either in 6C or 30C potencies, while high-potency medicines are usually prescribed by experienced and qualified homoeopaths.

The same remedy can be prescribed in different ways: for example, a single dose in a high-potency form or a remedy with a low dose but repeated frequently. The choice of how to administer the remedy depends on the nature of the illness and the individual needs of the patient. If a person has been ill for a considerable period of time and the body is physically damaged, repeated doses in a lower potency are better suited to stimulate the immune system, while a normally healthy person may respond quickly to a

single, high-potency remedy.

The more the remedy is diluted, the stronger it gets, as it possesses more energy and is, therefore, more capable of getting to the root cause of the problem, especially if it is a deep-seated one. It is fairly common for homoeopaths to use strengths such as 200C, 10M, etc. (M being used to denote 1,000C). Such high doses are usually used in the treatment of chronic disease, when it is said to act on the subtle energy level as well as the physical body.

Dilution also lessens the toxic effects of the drug, a matter of concern with the powerful and often dangerous drugs used in orthodox allopathic medicine. Since conventional drugs are prescribed for their individual capacities to act upon specific parts of the body, it follows that several different drugs might be prescribed to treat the various symptoms of one individual. The side-effects of these combinations are often unknown or not recognised. Homoeopathic medicine, on the other hand, prescribes a single medicine at a low dosage that will stimulate a person's immune and defence capacity and bring about an overall improvement in the person's health.

Homoeopathy And Skin Disorders

Skin disorders are viewed as the manifestation of some internal imbalance in the body. The skin is regarded as the outermost organ of the body, and skin troubles are believed to be the healthiest symptoms that a body can produce, as it heals from the inside out. The use of medicines that suppress these symptoms is, therefore, discouraged.

Note: Some skin conditions lend themselves to self-prescription, and remedies for these are listed in the following paragraphs. However, for chronic conditions an experienced homoeopathic practitioner should be consulted.

Boils And Abscesses

Which homoeopathic medicine is prescribed depends on the nature and development of the condition. If medicine is administered early, then the condition might be resolved before pus ever forms and, if given later, the medicines will help ripen the infection so that pus is eliminated speedily.

It is best to take or administer the medicine every three to four

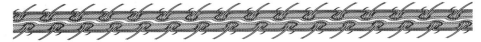

hours while redness, swelling and pain is most acute, and at least three doses should be tried before changing medicines in the event of there being no effect. Once definite signs of improvement are observed, treatment should be stopped for as long as the improvement continues. If the improvement stops or the condition regresses, then depending upon the symptoms, either the same remedy or a different remedy may be taken.

Some Useful Homoeopathic Remedies

Belladonna. This can be used during the initial stages of a localised boil where there is red, painful swelling, but little or no pus. Pains are throbbing or pounding. If Belladonna is ineffective after 24 hours of treatment, try the remedy below.

Hepar sulph. This is especially helpful before the pus has clearly formed, especially if the boil is very painful and tender to the touch. Throbbing and sharp pains accompanying a boil may indicate the need for this remedy.

Mercurius. Once the pus has formed, this remedy helps to bring the abscess to a head and speeds the drainage of pus. The type of boil suitable for this medicine is painful and aggravated by warmth.

Silica. Suitable for those boils and abscesses slow in healing, it is also helpful after a boil has been lanced or drained. The firm, red, cystic lumps that may persist after a boil has mostly healed often disappear after a dose of Silica 30C.

Arsenicum. This is useful for any stage of an abscess if there is great burning pain which can be relieved by warm applications.

Lachesis. To be chosen if the abscess or surrounding skin becomes purplish or blue.

Styes

These small abscesses, distinguished by their location in the eyelids, can be helped by any of the medicines referred to for the treatment of boils if any of the related symptoms indicate their use.

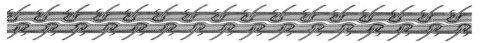

Some Useful Homoeopathic Remedies

Pulsatilla. This is one of the most commonly administered medicines for styes. The type of stye treated usually occurs on the upper eyelids, and comes to a head discharging yellow-green pus.

Hepar sulph. Effective when the stye is sensitive to the touch and is affected by cold applications and cool air. The pain from this stye is throbbing and sharp and may be relieved by warm applications.

Apis. For a painful stye which burns or stings, and also if the entire eyelid becomes red and swollen. Use the remedy if there is sensitivity and aggravation from heat and a definite relief from cold.

Graphites. Use this for a painful but less-tender stye, especially if there are crusts and sores on the eyelid and if a thick, yellow material is discharged.

Staphysagria. A recurring stye problem may be treated by this remedy, especially if the affected person suffers nervous exhaustion.

Impetigo

The remedy should be taken every four to six hours (for no longer than 48 hours) and stopped when improvement begins. Choose the medicine from the appropriate symptoms.

Some Useful Homoeopathic Remedies

Antimonium crudum. Useful for a condition where there is eruption and discharge, especially on the face, with thick, yellow crusts forming. Individual sores may run together into larger patches and increase in inflammation after cold bathing.

Graphites. For impetigo which is markedly scabby with oozing eruptions. Honey-coloured sores are common and prevalent around the mouth or nose.

Rhus tox. For very itchy conditions as well as stinging in the sores. Discharge from the sores is dark but translucent.

Mercurius. For open and deep sores with typical yellowish crusts. The discharge is pus-like with an unpleasant smell and possibly streaked with a little blood.

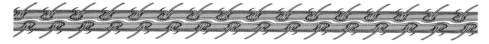

Hepar. Especially good if the sores are sensitive to the touch and cold, with soft and easily breakable scabs. The sores may bleed and be quite deep.

Arsenicum. For burning sores which feel raw and are relieved by warmth. The sores are dark and discharge a thin, watery liquid or pus.

Shingles

Use a homoeopathic treatment only in the absence of other significant health problems. If there are other significant health problems, see your practitioner. One dose of the selected medicine should be given every 12 hours for 36 hours, and should be stopped after any reaction is noted.

Some Useful Homoeopathic Remedies

Arsenicum. Useful for when the eruption burns intensely and there is relief in warmth but aggravation from cold air and cold applications.

Rhus tox. Use when there is intense itching and pain, the appearance of small blisters filled with a watery, yellow fluid and there is a lot of discomfort and restlessness at night.

Lachesis. Use this if the rash is dark red or has a purplish hue and the eruption is painful and sensitive when touched and is worse on the left side of the body.

Ranunculus bulbosus. Use when there is an attack of shingles involving the back or chest, and severe pain, especially in the ribs, which is worsened by touch, motion or lying on the rash as well as sudden exposure to heat or cold.

Mezereum. May be used when there are burning or sharp pains even after the eruption has gone. Patients are often chilly and sensitive to touch and cold.

Iris versicolor. Especially useful if the rash has affected the right side of the abdominal and chest region, and where there is the appearance of small blisters with dark points. The patient may have digestive upsets.

Other medicines for this condition include *Apis, Mercurius, Hepar sulph.* and *Sulphur.*

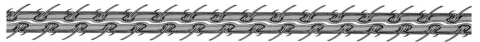

Warts

As this is a constitutional imbalance, it would be a very good idea to seek professional help.

Some Useful Homoeopathic Remedies

Causticum. May help with moist and jagged fleshy warts, especially on the fingernails or on the face, and warts with extra growth on them.

Dulcamara. May help with large, flat warts, especially prevalent on the backs of hands, fingers and on the face.

Antimonium crudum. For hard, horny and smooth-surfaced warts, especially on the hands.

Nitric acid. For warts on the face and lips. The warts may be soft, irregular and accompanied by sharp pains and bleeding. It is advisable to see your doctor with this type of wart.

Ringworm/Athlete's Foot

Choose a suitable remedy according to symptoms and administer a single dose once a day for three days. If the symptoms change, stop the medicine and allow recovery to take place.

Some Useful Homoeopathic Remedies

Sepia. Most useful for simple ringworm infections where there are circular, scaly patches, usually brown or reddish-brown. There may be itching and burning.

Tellurium. Use when the ringworm is more red than brown, with prominent rings. Small, itchy blisters releasing a thin liquid may appear on the rings.

Graphites. Use when there is a significant thick, honey-coloured discharge and the scales are thick.

Arsenicum. May help very dry ringworm with rough scales, a burning sensation and a discharge of clear liquid on scratching the area.

For ringworm of the scalp, all the above medicines are helpful.

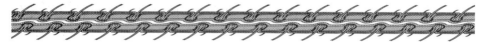

Candida (Yeast Infections)

If this is a recurrent problem, seek professional advice. Choose from the list below according to the most appropriate symptoms. Take twice daily for two to three days and stop when symptoms change.

Some Useful Homoeopathic Remedies

Belladonna. For when the skin is bright red and swollen with inflammation.

Chamomilla. For nappy rash with irritability.

Arsenicum. Use when the rash burns and itches. The skin might be raw and the watery fluid that is discharged is acrid and inflames the skin.

Graphites. For a honey-coloured discharge, and when raw areas become encrusted. The skin may, however, appear just dry, rough and cracked.

Hepar. Use when there is a secondary bacterial infection and pimples and pus forms on raw areas which smell unpleasant. There will be extreme tenderness of the inflamed parts.

When there are thrush infections of the mouth, the following remedies are suggested:

Borax. The best remedy to try initially if symptoms do not indicate any of the others. There may be sores on the mucous membranes, dryness in the mouth, a little swelling and bleeding.

Mercurius. Use when the mouth is sore and inflamed and emits an unpleasant odour; there is considerable salivation, the gums are soft and bleed easily and may be streaked with white lines; the tongue is puffy and coated either with a black, white or dirty-yellow colour.

Hydrastis. For a large amount of thick mucus in the mouth and on the tongue, which experiences a burning sensation.

Eczema

This is a chronic and deep-seated condition, and so consultation with a skilled homoeopathic practitioner is strongly advised to determine individual diagnosis and remedies.

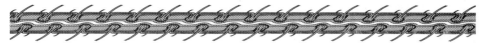

Hives

If this is recurrent, seek professional advice.

Some Useful Homoeopathic Remedies

Apis. The most likely medicine for the condition, where the hives are intensely itchy and aggravated by warmth, and may come out during perspiration and after exercise. The remedy is particularly helpful for hives which cause swelling around the eyes, and when hives look swollen and waterlogged.

Urtica urens (stinging nettle). This may be considered when the symptoms are similar to those needing Apis and are especially prevalent after strenuous exercise.

Rhus tox. Use this if the condition seems to be caused by rubbing, scratching or wetness, and is much worse at night, causing restlessness.

Psoriasis

Psoriasis should be treated by an experienced homoeopathic practitioner.

Acne

Acne should be treated by an experienced homoeopathic practitioner.

Some Useful Homoeopathic Remedies

Kali bichromicum. Use this for chronic acne.

Sulphur. Use this for inflamed and infected pustules.

Psorinum. Use this for itchy infections.

Bruises

Some Useful Homoeopathic Remedies

Arnica oil. Rubbing this on to the affected area may be helpful.

Arnica cream or ointment. Use this **only** if the skin is unbroken. It is better to take Arnica internally if it is broken.

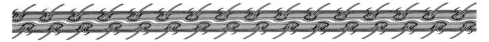

A Conversation With A Homoeopathic Practitioner

Q. What is the goal of homoeopathic treatment?
A. The goal is to get you to a level of health, balance and freedom from limitations so that you eventually need only very infrequent medication.

Q. Why do homoeopaths ask so many questions?
A. Constitutional homoeopathy does not treat specific diseases as such, but treats individuals. Hence a detailed understanding of the patient is fundamental to making a correct prescription.

The homoeopath must attempt an almost impossible task – that of coming quickly to a complete understanding of an individual. The questioning process is essential for forming and developing this understanding.

The homoeopath needs to be an acute listener and observer – their job is primarily to get your symptom picture and to match this to a remedy. They want to hear your story and will listen sympathetically, without making any value judgements. To match a remedy to an individual, the homoeopath must know all the person's limitations: this includes mental, emotional and physical levels, and such aspects as general energy, effects of environment, and causative factors.

Q. How many appointments are necessary?
A. In the beginning (that is, in the first six months), visits may be more frequent and will taper off as you become healthier. We feel we need to see you initially more frequently (follow-up appointments are usually every four to six weeks in the beginning) to work with you and evaluate your progress. Yet we are not insensitive to the cost of treatment, and do not wish to make this a burden. A happy medium can be reached.

If a remedy has acted curatively, even in deep and complex cases, after the initial follow-up we may not need to see you for some time. This is because the remedy has brought your system into balance and, in our experience, this state can last for a long time. We also need to wait until the next 'remedy picture' comes up clearly. This is the time to have a renewed faith in your body's healing abilities.

Q. How can I be involved?
A. You don't have to believe in homoeopathic remedies in order for them to work (we treat babies and there are homoeopathic vets). But to select

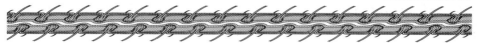

the correct remedy and for the treatment to continue to act, your co-operation and commitment is necessary. You can help by:

- Noting any changes after you take the remedy – keeping a weekly journal can be helpful for bringing to your follow-up consultations. Please note general changes as well as specific ones.
- Being clear and complete about your symptoms on all levels.
- A commitment to a long-term process and perspective is really a commitment to your long-term well-being.
- Above all, communicating any concerns or questions you may have. We are always trying to find better ways of helping you and welcome your comments.

Q. How do homoeopaths evaluate a curative response?
A. Homoeopaths have, through over 170 years of experience, developed sophisticated means of evaluating curative responses and have established laws and principles of cure.

On a simpler level, you want to see the problems you have come with clear up, and they should. Always keep in mind that ours is a total perspective on you and we want to see overall improvements as well as specific ones. You also have to see improvement in the context of the amount of stress in your life. So improvements will occur on physical, emotional and mental levels, and in general energy. Observe and report these general changes as well as specific ones.

Q. How long does treatment take?
A. This is a difficult question to answer, but after several interviews the homoeopath is better able to give you an idea of this. In simpler problems and in acute situations, results can begin quickly and dramatically.

For a small percentage of very healthy individuals, one or two treatments may be all that is needed to stabilise the system for years at a stretch, but such an ideal would, for most people, be an unrealistic expectation.

Q. Should I come back after I am feeling better?
A. The four to six week follow-up is important to return for. After you are feeling consistently better, we would like to see you for regular check-ups to prevent future problems. Usually, this is at four to six month intervals.

Q. Where are the remedies from?
A. We either have your remedy available at the clinic and will dispense it, the cost usually being included in your consultation fee, or we shall refer you to a convenient homoeopathic pharmacy.

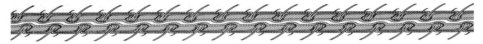

There are over 2,000 remedies in use, and these are prepared in established homoeopathic pharmacies, but most homoeopathic prescriptions are made from a narrower range of 200 to 300 remedies.

For more information about specific remedies, their origin and nature, refer to the reading list at the end of this guide.

Q. How can a few doses do anything or last a long time?

A. The remedies are highly potent – they are prepared in what is called a potentised dilution and are dropped on to tiny lactose granules or as powders, tablets, pillules or liquid. They simply catalyse, or trigger, a response by the body on an energetic level, rather than effect chemical change. So, ultimately, what works better after the remedy is taken is your own regulating system. The remedy helps the body to develop a natural, positive momentum which continues to gain strength and eliminate disease.

Should you want to gain a more in-depth understanding of this fascinating and profound process, refer to the *Headway Lifeguide* on *Homoeopathy* or to any of the introductory books on the reading list.

Q. Is there any advice about diet and lifestyle?

A. The homoeopath doesn't always give advice about lifestyle and diet. A good diet is, of course, essential for a healthy body. Any advice about diet and exercise is tailored to the individual's own needs in terms of their illness, age, and various environmental factors. This is because we always want to see clearly whether the homoeopathic remedy alone is working. Also we believe that when the organism is healthy, an imbalanced lifestyle will diminish and positive changes will permeate all aspects of your life. There may be obvious 'obstacles to cure' in your life or environment which the homoeopath will discuss with you.

Q. Can homoeopathy work in more complex or chronic cases, and how long does it take?

A. In more complex cases, homoeopathic treatment is 'like peeling away the layers of an onion'. Briefly, this means that we build up layers of symptoms, or pathology, as a response to certain stresses we go through life. These 'layers' are laid down and can be 'peeled' away effectively with homoeopathic remedies. During treatment, old sets of symptoms may come up (but because with each successive remedy you are healthier, they will not be as severe as in the past). A recurrence of an old set of symptoms may be the indication for a new remedy to be given. Even some hereditary tendencies can be eliminated with homoeopathy.

So in deep or chronic problems, the curative process may be gradual and consultations more frequent.

Q. What happens if the symptoms seem to return?

A. If you had a good curative response to a remedy and then after, say, two to six months (or at any time) a relapse seems to occur, we usually recommend waiting a few days to see if your system re-balances itself. If any severe symptoms develop, do not wait. If the symptoms persist after a week, then a repeat of the remedy may be necessary. If so, another appointment would be needed.

Do not get disappointed or discouraged at this point and feel that homoeopathy is not working for you – this is just a phase of getting you to a consistently good state of health.

This situation may mean a new remedy is indicated as a 'layer' of symptoms from the past comes up and needs to be treated.

Q. What will interfere with the remedy working?

A. The major interfering factors are camphor products and highly aromatic essential oils, such as peppermint and menthol. There are also certain therapies that can interfere, such as chemical therapies (natural or otherwise), high-potency vitamins, very intensive exercise programmes, and certain dental procedures. It is not usually a good idea to have acupuncture during a course of homoeopathic treatment, as acupuncture may interfere with the flow of energy or the 'vital force'.

We have found that massage, mild chiropractic and osteopathic treatments and certain gentle therapies or medications do not interfere with homoeopathy.

If you are considering any other therapy, consult your homoeopath first.

It is also best to avoid, or at least greatly reduce, the intake of coffee and other caffeine drinks.

Q. Can a wrong remedy be given and what are the effects?

A. Much as we try to match the correct remedy, we do not always achieve 100 per cent accuracy. If appropriately used, homoeopathic treatment, however, should produce no side-effects from the remedies.

Generally speaking, either nothing changes or the true symptom picture will become even clearer and the right remedy is more obvious.

It can take several interviews for a homoeopath to get an accurate picture of the totality of your symptoms and an essential understanding of this to select the right remedy. Of course, the clearer and more in touch you are with yourself, the easier this task becomes.

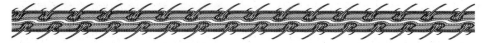

Q. What about seeing a GP?

A. Homoeopathy is complementary to the health care that is available. We recommend that you should maintain your relationship with your doctor, especially for routine needs and emergencies. Your GP will also arrange for you to have any blood tests or X-rays, etc. or refer you to a consultant.

Q. What about acute problems?

A. Homoeopathic remedies can treat acute problems, such as flu and stomach upsets, and even help the body heal after injuries and falls. If you are already having homoeopathic treatment, mild illnesses will often clear up on their own, but if you are unsure or the symptoms are getting stronger, please phone for advice. If your symptoms are severe, phone immediately. If necessary contact your GP.

If you are involved in an accident or emergency, you should go to your nearest casualty department for treatment and then phone to see if a homoeopathic remedy is also indicated.

Finding A Practitioner

A register of doctors who have taken a postgraduate course is maintained by the Faculty of Homoeopathy, c/o Royal London Homoeopathic Hospital, Great Ormond Street, London, WC1N 3HR. For a list of registered homoeopaths, write to The Society of Homoeopaths, 2 Artizan Road, Northampton, NN1 4HU.

Further Reading

Homoeopathy: Headway Lifeguides by Beth MacEoin
    (Hodder & Stoughton)
Homoeopathy for Emergencies by Phyllis Speight (C W Daniels)
The Complete Homoeopathy Handbook: A Guide to Everyday Health Care
    by Miranda Castro (Macmillan)
*The Family Guide to Homoeopathy: The Safe Form of Medicine for the
    Future* by Andrew Lockie (Elm Tree Books)
Homoeopathy, Medicine for the New Man by George Vithoulkas
    (Thorsons)
Everybody's Guide to Homoeopathic Medicines by Stephen Cummings
    and Dana Ullman (Gollancz)
Homoeopathy: Medicine for the 21st Century by Dana Ullman
    (Thorsons)

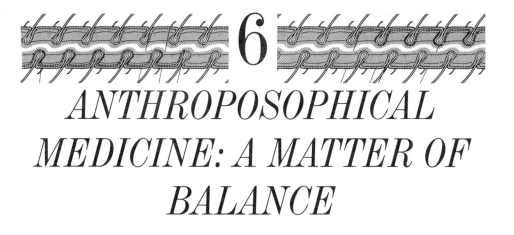

ANTHROPOSOPHICAL MEDICINE: A MATTER OF BALANCE

Anthroposophical medicine is founded on the view that the functioning of life cannot be purely explained by physical or chemical processes. Rather, there is a spiritual aspect that is vital to consider when treating an illness. This way of thinking was first propounded by Rudolf Steiner, an Austrian scientist and philosopher, in the late nineteenth and early twentieth centuries, and was put into practice by a group of doctors in Europe in the 1920s.

This medical system is seen by its advocates to be an extension of the practices and ideals of conventional medicine, and is not simply an 'alternative' therapy, such as homoeopathy and acupuncture. Steiner recognised the achievements of natural science and the progress of medical and surgical techniques, all based on the assumption that illness represents a physical breakdown in the body. Yet he felt that this was too limited an approach to take. His ideas, outlined first in his fundamental work, *The Philosophy of Freedom,* saw the nature of man as being one of soul and spirit as well as body. Steiner was also interested in a renewal of the arts, and founded a new art of movement, *eurhythmy,* which was later incorporated into his approach to therapy.

Steiner was not a medically trained doctor and, indeed, was not drawn into the medical aspects of his philosophy until late in his life. His role was that of a consultant, not only to the medical profession, but also to other vocational fields. He was approached by teachers of able-bodied and handicapped children, architects and farmers interested in the principles of anthroposophy. In the sphere of medicine, Steiner worked with doctors who saw that anthroposophy could make a real contribution to medical practice, and with the close collaboration of the physician, Dr Ita Wegman, the foundation for the new medicine was laid.

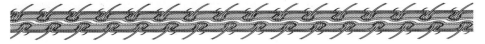

The Principles Of The Medicine

As anthroposophical medicine is considered to be an extension rather than an alternative to conventional *(allopathic)* medicine, it is pertinent to consider the relationship between the two. Conventional medicine is based on physical experiment and observation guided by hypotheses which have to be tangible and measurable. This means that, in the view of those who adhere simply to conventional medical practices, any non-tangible realities do not exist or are not accessible to investigation. This assumption has the consequence that all living, emotional and mental aspects of existence must finally be reduced to physical ends. *Reductionism*, seeing the essentials of life in the smallest terms, is a fundamental tenet of conventional medicine, and one which is challenged by anthroposophical medicine.

Anthroposophical medicine sees the functioning of life as more than just a physical entity and argues, in particular, that disciplined thought need not be confined to physical realities and, indeed, if this were so, then a good deal of higher mathematics would not exist. Steiner considered that there was more to the theory of why life functioned than purely physical and material explanations. He thought that there were aspects such as the spirit and the soul, which were equally important but had been disregarded because they were seen to be immeasurable.

The Four Aspects Of A Human Person

In addition to the physical body, three other elements are present which complete the picture of the human being. In anthroposophical terms, they are called the *etheric body*, the *astral body* and the *ego*. These elements are common to us all, but cannot be perceived by the physical senses. Put simply, the etheric body is that which is concerned with growth and replenishment; the astral body represents emotions; and the ego, an individual spiritual core which man alone possesses.

The Etheric Body

This is best described as the force which governs the vitality of the physical body. This is the *life element* of the body, and we can see that after death, when only the physical body is left, the body

begins to decay under the influence of physical laws.

The etheric body is responsible for building the physical parts of the body into a whole, and in maintaining this living structure by continuous repairing and restructuring. It is the source of a natural tendency to recover from less serious ailments without additional medical help. In short, it constantly fights against death and decay.

The Astral Body

This is the soul element that is common to animals and human beings, and is what differentiates them from the plant kingdom. Consciousness of the physical world and instinct are qualities associated with the astral body; we are aware of emotions and pain not only on a physical level, but also on an inner level of feeling and thought, a level which cannot be measured tangibly but is still very much there. This is where the main difference between anthroposophical and conventional doctors is to be found. The former consider the soul element as much as the physical element; the latter are concerned primarily with the physical aspect. Anthroposophical practitioners see life as a growth process of the soul and as spiritual development; crises are often seen as positive phases in this development.

The astral body has a *catabolic* (breaking down) effect on the human body, and so has an opposite effect to the etheric body, which is constantly endeavouring to build and repair. So, good health prevails as long as the destructive process, due to the actions of the astral body, are held in check and in equilibrium by the replenishing and building force of the etheric body. When there is an imbalance between the two, disease will result.

The Ego

Present only in human beings, this is an additional level of consciousness that can be described as *self-consciousness*. It comprises the ability to think and an awareness of being autonomous. So humans are able to refrain from instinctive behaviour if their reasoning leads them to believe that it is better to do so, a quality that is not present in animals. This spirit (or *ego*) has a dual effect on the physical body, as it works on the etheric body in its anabolic activity and with the astral body in its catabolic activity.

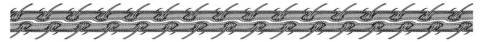

The Anthroposophical View Of Illness

Illness is considered in terms of the interrelationship between the ego, the astral body, the etheric body and the physical body. The aim is to influence the activity of one or more of these elements so as to restore an individual balance and, therefore, health. The anthroposophical view of bodily functions must be understood, as it explains how illness is diagnosed and treated.

It is thought that the four aspects of man (the physical or mineral body, the etheric or life body, the astral or sentient body and the ego) are connected to each other and relate to each other in different ways in the different areas of the human body and its organ systems. For instance, in the nerve–sense system with a central focus in the senses, we find little evidence of vitality, regeneration and movement; the nerve tissue is extremely vulnerable and easily damaged if oxygen and other nutrients are witheld. Therefore, the etheric forces must be weakly connected to these organs, and the astral organisation expresses itself directly in a catabolic way: *sentient* functions (thought, perception, consciousness) find their instrument primarily in the nerve–sense system, reflex organisation and (embodied in anabolic functions also) autonomic nervous system. Inasfar as the ego finds expression in self-consciousness, it uses the nerve–sense system.

In the opposite, *anabolic,* function of the body, the life-bringing forces of the etheric body are much more connected to the physical body. We find a wealth of vitality, often exuberant growth activity, in many glandular organs, the reproductive organs and many of the main organs of the digestive tract (liver, pancreas, etc.). The muscles of our limbs are also full of life and voluntary movement: this suggests a contribution of the sentient body and ego within these organ systems, but less 'conscious' as found in the nerve–sense system. (Anabolic serves catabolic in the metabolic–limb system, whilst catabolic overrules anabolic in the nerve–sense system.)

So we can say that in the nerve–sense organisation, life is pushed back to the brink of death/dying, and enables consciousness to arise; in the metabolic and limb system, life is present and embued by sentient directives; what holds the delicate balance continuously is the rhythmical organisation: in its purest, functional form visible in the breathing and circulation – functions wherein a rhythym maintains a constantly changing balance

between *systole* (contraction, consciousness enhancing) and *distole* (relaxation, regeneration bringing).

Within this functional system the contrasting nerve–sense system in its primary catabolic activity, and the metabolic limb system, with its regenerating potential, interpenetrate and balance. Such an artistic view of the functional system of the human body enables the anthroposophical practitioner to relate anatomical, physiological aspects to psychological and spiritual aspects in an often very direct way. Dis-ease results from an imbalance of the described systems and the four aspects working in them. Different methods can be used to restore such imbalances.

It is thought that the four aspects of man, the physical, etheric and astral bodies, and the ego, are connected to each other by means of three interpenetrating bodily systems – the metabolic limb, the nerve–sense system, and the rhythmic system.

The *metabolic limb system* is governed mainly by the physical and etheric bodies, and regulates the digestive and excretory processes and the glandular system as well as restoring and rebuilding the body. Organs such as the liver, the digestive tracts and the muscles are prominent.

The *nerve–sense system* is influenced mainly by the ego and the astral body controlling conscious processes, such as thought and perception. This system is in control during the daytime when we are awake, and gives way to the metabolic limb system during sleeping hours to allow the body to be replenished. The nerve–sense system incorporates the nerves, the spinal cord, the brain and the sense organs, and activity is concentrated mainly in the head.

Between the two systems lies the *rhythmic system*. It is formed by the alternation of the other two systems and controls processes, such as circulation and breathing. It is centred on the region of the chest and functions through the heart, lungs and circulatory system. Within this system, the contrasting nerves and senses and the metabolic functions interpenetrate and produce all bodily rhythms. In short, the rhythmic system helps keep the nerve system and the metabolic limb system in a state of balance.

In anthroposophical medicine, illnesses are divided into two main groups: *inflammatory* (or feverish) and *degenerative* (or hardening). Inflammatory diseases are thought to arise when the person's metabolic and digestive system becomes too strong, leading to an excess of warmth and fluid. These include many childhood disorders, such as measles and chicken-pox. Degenerative diseases are said to arise from the hardening effect of the astral body and ego on the nerve–sense system and include conditions such as cancer and hardening of the arteries.

As illness is the result of an imbalance between the nerve–sense system and the metabolic limb system, it follows that a cure can only be effected when the balance is restored. The practitioner will use different methods to achieve this.

Types Of Treatment

Remedies

Most of the medicines come from mainly plant or mineral sources, but some come from animals; special attention is paid to the particular qualities of the origin of the medicine. Remedies are often based on life processes in nature which are similar to those in the human organism. Steiner believed that many natural substances were related to aspects of physical health, for example that the seven metals – lead, tin, iron, copper, gold, mercury and silver – corresponded to certain bodily organs. So an anthroposophical doctor might prescribe a 'potentised' remedy or ointment made from tin for a patient with liver problems or, perhaps, copper for kidney regulation. Depending on individual circumstances and the nature of the problem, medicines may be prescribed either in material doses or in potentised ones.

Artistic Therapies

It is thought that much illness derives from the individual's estrangement from his own creative capacity, and that fundamental healing can only take place if this is restored. Activities, such as music, painting, sculpture and architecture, help in the healing process and are often recommended within an integrated treatment. Painting is thought to be an expression of the astral in the etheric level, while sculpture is a manifestation of the etheric level in the physical body.

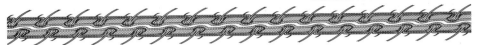

Eurhythmy

This 'art of movement' devised by Steiner has also been called *visible speech* and *visible music*. It aims to restore a healthy, balanced relationship between the soul and the physical body, and works towards a reunion of the patient's thoughts, feelings and actions. The art consists of bodily movements and gestures which are related to the vowel and consonant sounds that are made when speaking. The sounds of speech are formed by movements of the larynx, lips, teeth and tongue in conjunction with the flow of breath. The effects of therapeutic eurhythmy, during which rhythmical bodily movements are performed in harmony with the rhythm of the spoken word, include a greater appreciation of rhythm and suppleness.

Hydrotherapy And Massage

Water is the one medium that we have all experienced before birth in the womb and is, therefore, considered by practitioners to play a special role in the healing process. History illustrates the value placed on therapeutic baths by ancient civilisations and in the development of spa towns, many of which are still in existence today.

Baths with certain essential oils are helpful for the alleviation of circulatory and muscular problems, and can distribute warmth where it may be lacking as a result of illness.

The therapeutic value of massage is well known. Anthroposophical medicine has developed a particular kind of massage technique known as *rhythmic massage,* which aims to balance the etheric force with the tension created by the astral influence. This is done by encouraging regularity in breathing and heart action, and the other natural cycles in order to harmonise the workings of bodily functions.

Anthroposophical Medicine And Skin Disorders

Anthroposophical medicine views the skin as a vital part of the immune system, effective against bacteria and viruses, only breached when the skin is damaged or weakened. The skin has many qualities associated with the nerve–sense system, as it is sensitive to temperature and pain. It is, therefore, regarded as an extensive sense organ. Skin disorders occur when the

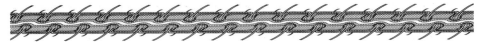

breaking-down quality (catabolic) of the nerve–sense system is out of balance with the life force (anabolic) quality of the metabolic system.

Deep in the layers of the skin there is close contact with the nerve capillaries and here skin cells reproduce rapidly. Over a period of time, these new skin cells progress upwards through the layers of the skin and lose their capacity to divide and form new skin cells. Instead, part of the skin cells fills with a protein called keratin. This protein has the effect of hardening the skin cells and the cells die in reaching the outermost layers of the skin, remaining hard because of the keratin. It is these dead, hard skin cells which provide a tough, protective barrier against the outer world. The health of the skin depends on maintaining the balance between the vital reproductive activity of the deeper layers and the deadening process nearer the surface. In anthroposophical medicine, when this balance between the actions of the nerve sense (deadening) and the metabolic (life force) systems is breached, skin problems occur.

Eczema provides a good example of this. When the life or metabolic processes predominate, this is when the inflammatory and wet phase of eczema prevails. The skin can become infected as there is no longer a protective layer of hardened cells. Yet when the nerve–sense system dominates and there is too much deadening of the cells, this shows up in the dry, scaly phase of eczema.

A Conversation With An Anthroposophical Practitioner

Q. Where do you place eczema in the anthroposophical system?
A. Eczema is an obvious imbalance between the metabolic organisation (leading to inflammation), and the nerve–sense system (which brings the form aspect): in eczema the metabolic dominates and the skin starts to digest itself exuberantly, leading to the wet, cracked, often infected and inflamed, picture of eczema. More often than not, the cause is therefore to be found in the metabolic digestive system, the symptoms of which are to be found in the skin itself.

Q. What is the basis of treatment?

A. If the metabolic predominates, as it does in the inflammatory stage of eczema, the formative nerve–sense system needs reinforcing. We often use bitter and astringent remedies to be taken by mouth: extracts of dandelion root and gentian root. If the form aspect (sense-nerve system) dominates and a hardening and thickening of the skin takes place, we turn to remedies to restore normal form: silica could be used but also potentised tin. With regard to external applications, oak bark ointment or antimony ointment would be used. Of course diet should be taken into account.

Q. What about psoriasis?

A. Psoriasis is in my experience more difficult to treat. Both metabolic/inflammatory and nerve–sense system/hardening take place at the same time in psoriasis. The skin appears both young and red as well as old and flaky. Once again, diet is of utmost importance in the long-term management of this condition. Often the hardening predominates and sulphur baths could aid in stimulating the anabolic forces. External applications in the form of ointments are also used. The anabolic functions of the liver can be enhanced by compresses of yarrow to the liver area.

Q. What is the anthroposophical view in skin infections?

A. Skin infections occur when the host boundaries are weakened. The vitality (etheric forces) of the body as a whole needs addressing and strengthening. Local treatment, for instance calendula lotion or ointment, can be used. Primarily, however, one should ask why the boundaries are weakened.

Finding A Practitioner

Anthroposophical practitioners are qualified medical doctors who have then taken a further postgraduate course recognised by the Anthroposophical Medical Association in Britain. Some may be found working in the NHS, although others work privately or in the Rudolf Steiner schools and homes for children. Residential treatment in certain private clinics is also available.

Consultations are very much like seeing a GP, except that there will be additional details and questions about, for example, lifestyle and emotional conditions. Diagnosis is made in the same

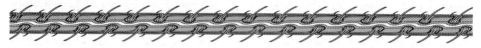

way as a GP, but treatment is prescribed depending on the individual characteristics of the patient. Treatment ranges from conventional to herbal or homoeopathic remedies. Practitioners may try and bring about long-term changes, in addition to alleviating symptoms, by prescribing eurhythmy or an art therapy in order to sort out an underlying imbalance, and might send a patient to a specialist.

The Anthroposophical Medical Association maintains a register of members. It is based at the Park Attwood Therapeutic Centre, Trimpley, Bewdley, Worcestershire, DY12 1RE.

Further Reading

Anthroposophical Medicine by Dr M. Evans and I. Roger (Thorsons)
Anthroposophical Medicine and Its Remedies by Otto Wolf (Weleda Ag)
Rudolf Steiner: Scientist of the Invisible by A.P. Shepherd (Floris Books)

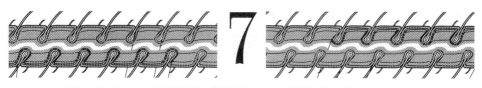

7

AROMATHERAPY: MORE THAN JUST SCENTING THE SKIN

Aromatherapy uses plants and their oils for healing and for medicine. Although the term itself was not coined until the twentieth century, aromatherapy has a long and distinguished tradition. Records dating back to at least 2000 BC make mention of such techniques.

The Bible refers to the use of plants and their oils for the treatment of illnesses, and it is well known that the Egyptians used essential oils for embalming their dead, and as cosmetics. The Egyptians are considered to have developed the technique of aromatherapy into an art form, and the botanical gardens of Egypt were wondrous to behold, containing rare plants collected from India and China. Indeed, so skilled did the Egyptian priests and priestesses become, that physicians came from all over the world to study medicine in Egypt.

Aromatic oils were used extensively in China, too. The earliest written document describing aromatic techniques is Chinese, and dates back to 1000–700 BC. In ancient China, herbal medicine was used in conjunction with acupuncture and massage as the principal form of health care.

To the Greeks, aromatics were part of their everyday life: sweet incense was burnt in the temples and during state ceremonies, and food and wine was extensively scented. Hippocrates, the 'Father of Medicine', recommended the taking of a daily aromatic bath and claimed that a scented massage would prolong life.

The Arab peoples in their explorations searched for, and discovered, many aromatic fragrances. The Far East yielded sandalwood, cassia, camphor, nutmeg, myrrh and cloves, which were used in medicine and perfumery. It was the Arab physician, Abu Ibn Sina, known in the West as Avicenna, who is credited with perfecting the process of the distillation of the essential oils, a method so advanced that the apparatus for it has changed very little in 900 years.

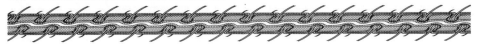

Herbs such as fennel and parsley, were introduced into England by conquering legions of Roman soldiers and, later, the twelfth century saw the introduction of aromatic oils into England brought by crusading knights on their way back from the Holy Land. More importantly, they brought with them the knowledge of how to distil the oils.

The medieval period saw an increase in the use of oils in medicine and perfumery. Glove makers used to perfume their wares with oils to mask the body odour of the wearer, and it was a well-observed fact in the Middle Ages that during times of cholera and other epidemics, the perfumers rarely succumbed. This was mainly because nearly all essential oils are antiseptics.

The Renaissance gave impetus to the study of medicine and, in the sixteenth and seventeenth centuries, essential oils were widely used as antiseptics, perfumes and medicines, and new plant species were available as a result of the opening up of America to Europe through colonisation. But as chemistry began to flourish as a discipline, plant substances were increasingly synthesised in the laboratory, and these chemical copies, which did not have the same medicinal properties as the original essential oils, took over from natural essential oils, being cheaper to manufacture.

In the twentieth century, however, there has been marked revival of interest in natural treatments, with a corresponding demand for genuine essential oils. This revival was pioneered by Professor Rene Gattefosse who discovered by accident the remarkable healing power of lavender oil when he burnt his hand and plunged it into the nearest liquid, which happened to be the essential oil of lavender. On seeing how quickly his hand healed without leaving a scar, Gattefosse went on to research further the effects of essential oils, and treated many soldiers wounded in the First World War. It was he who coined the word *aromatherapy*. The discipline was further developed by a French physician, Dr Jean Valnet, and a French biochemist, Marguerite Maury, and the technique is now practised by many enthusiasts.

Aromatherapy At Work

Aromatherapy is a holistic therapy which aims to deal with the patient not only on a physical level, but also mentally, emotionally and spiritually. The essential oils are used to restore equilibrium on all levels, and are even used to prevent ill health and to promote well-being.

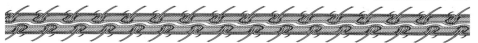

The Use Of Essential Oils

Essential oils are found in all plants and herbs. They are what gives fragrance to flowers, such as rose or lavender, or flavour to herbs, such as cinnamon or ginger. Oil can be extracted from any part of the plant – from petals and leaves, roots, seeds and rinds.

Most oils are extracted through a process known as *steam distillation*, in which steam is passed under pressure through the plant material. The heat causes the release and evaporation of the oil, which then passes through a water cooler where it turns back into liquid and is then collected. A more recent development is *vacuum distillation*, which works by reducing air pressure inside the sealed apparatus allowing distillation at much lower temperatures. This is significant because it preserves the delicate flower fragrances more successfully. Oils from citrus fruits are found in the outer rind of the fruits, so simple pressure is applied to extract the oils, a technique known as *expression*.

These details are not only of academic interest. They have environmental implications, too. Many oils on the market are not as pure or as natural as they are made out to be. Many contain adulterants to enhance the aroma or to dilute the oil, while other extraction processes leave behind pesticide residues or chemical solvents from the process itself. Aromatherapists stress the importance of purely extracted essential oils for the treatment to be as effective as possible.

Aromatic oils are often thought to be the 'life-force' of the plants in which they are found, and their effect on the human body is the basis of aromatherapy. Apart from promoting a state of well-being and harmony, particular oils have specific therapeutic properties. Nearly all essential oils tend to be powerful antiseptics, which destroy bacteria and viruses. They promote the holistic ideal by stimulating the immune system, thereby encouraging the body to resist disease, as well as improving the circulatory system, relieving pain and reducing fluid retention.

Chemically, essential oils are complex substances, and the ways in which they exercise their effects on the body are similarly complicated. The oils contain, in many cases, up to 100 chemical constituents, and it is evident that each constituent, however minor, performs some vital function. The reactions between these constituents and their component molecules give the oil its therapeutic value, which is why synthetic equivalents can never be equally effective.

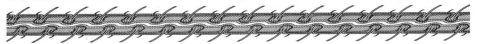

Further, there is evidence to suggest that some essential oils have a high electrical resistance, and that this quality may help in the treatment of problems where the electrical resistance of cells is low.

It is not always possible to discern how a particular oil has a particular therapeutic effect. Aromatherapy often works on the basis of empiricism: that which works, works and will not be rejected in the absence of scientific proof.

Touch And Smell

A partial explanation of how aromatherapy works is provided when we consider the workings of our senses of smell and touch. As its name suggests, aromatherapy is concerned with aroma, or odour, which induces an effect on the human body. This is because our sense of smell works on a subconscious level, and smell can affect emotional behaviour. Olfactory nerves (nerves involved in the sense of smell) affect memory and thought. Different odours can stimulate the brain and evoke images or feelings associated with that particular smell; aromatherapy uses this in dealing with the mental and emotional aspects of healing. Different smells are used to stimulate or relax the patient as the need may be.

The sense of touch is one of the most important ways through which a new human being adjusts itself to the world, and studies have shown that babies in incubators who are regularly held and fondled by their parents make a speedier recovery in terms of their mental and physical development. Since touching is so essential for good health, it can be seen how important massage is to aromatherapy. The pleasurable sensation of being touched induces feelings of being loved and cared for, which is vital for emotional well-being.

Massage also confers physical benefits on the recipient – stimulating the immune system, reducing high blood pressure and improving circulation of the blood and lymphatic systems, to name but a few. Massage can also reduce muscular tension or swelling, as well as relieving pain in the muscles and joints. These physical effects aid relaxation, which is so important in the healing process and contributes to the alleviation of psychological tension and frayed emotions.

Aromatherapy can also treat specific problem areas. Some major organs of the body, such as the large intestine, are accessible to

massage, while organs such as the liver and kidneys, which are
more internally placed, can be influenced by massaging the area of
the body under which they are situated. It is believed that such
organs can be aided through stimulating the nerves and increasing
the local blood supply. Some aromatherapists use pressure point
techniques, as in reflexology and acupressure, for a more
sophisticated and specific massage therapy. Massage with essential
oils is applied to the pressure points to stimulate internal organs.

However, massage is not the only aromatherapeutic technique.
An aromatic bath is a pleasurable way of enjoying the benefits of
essential oils. Hot water opens sores and helps the body to absorb
the oils more quickly. Baths can also alleviate the effects of stress,
as well as relieving muscular pain and skin conditions. Essential
oils are effective, too, when inhaled. Their aromatic molecules
reach the lungs and are diffused across the air sacs. They
eventually arrive in the bloodstream from where they exercise
their therapeutic effects.

Stress Relief

Aromatherapy is particularly effective in dealing with stress and
stress-related disorders. 'Stress' is a term which encompasses a
wide spectrum of problems and symptoms which, in turn, can lead
to more serious illnesses. Aromatherapy, in helping to relax the
patient and by reducing stress, may actually help to prevent such
conditions. Stress-related disorders, such as digestive problems,
acne and other skin problems, can be treated by aromatherapy. As
stress is reduced, there is a corresponding improvement in sleep
patterns and energy levels.

Skin Disorders

Healthy skin reflects a healthy body, and a blemished or flaking
skin is often the result of some internal disorder. So it is vital to
take account of factors such as diet and lifestyle when considering
the condition of the skin. Imperfect skin can also be due to
hereditary causes, and eczema and psoriasis and even hay fever
may leave the sufferer with blemished skin.

From a practical point of view, aromatherapy can deal with skin
problems through the use of good skin care products which
contain essential oils for the particular condition. Care of the skin

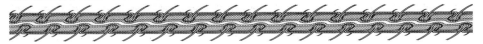

involves regular washing with a mild pH-balanced soap or cleanser and toning and moisturising with, if possible, natural and gentle products. The type of product should be suited to the particular skin type. Essential oils can be added to lotions, or homemade lotions containing the oils can be made for everyday skin care.

Eczema And Dermatitis

Both diseases have broadly similar symptoms, characterised by inflammation, swelling and itchy rashes, often leading to blisters and weeping scabs. The skin is often flaky, and patches of skin may be blotchy. The essential oils considered to be the most appropriate for these problems are fennel, camomile, geranium, sandalwood, hyssop, juniper and lavender.

There are many self-help measures that can be taken. Simple application of the essential oil in a suitable carrier is beneficial. If the eczema is dry, then calendula oil is recommended as a carrier, while if the eczema is moist, a carrier lotion is preferred. Twelve drops added to 50 ml of the oil or lotion and applied to the affected area every morning or night will relieve the eczema. It depends on the individual as to which oil is the most beneficial, and it is advisable to visit a therapist who can further advise on the best method of skin care. Products containing lanolin are to be avoided as it is a frequent cause of allergy, as are most dairy products. Infusions made with calendula or camomile sprayed on to the face will act as a soothing, cooling remedy.

Acne

Acne is a common skin condition occurring especially around puberty and the menopause, and is due to hormonal imbalances. Stress and anxiety can also contribute to the problem.

As well as specific aromatherapeutic treatment, it is essential that diet, exercise, fresh air and cleanliness are included as part of the programme. Regular and meticulous cleansing, toning and moisturising are a prerequisite for the oils to be effective. Oils especially appropriate for acne include calendula, camomile, juniper, lavender, mint, myrrh, myrtle, neroli, palmarosa, tea tree and thyme.

A typical treatment for normal skin would be to mix together 50 ml soya oil, 6 drops wheatgerm oil and 10 drops of the chosen essential oil. For extra-sensitive skin, mix together 25 ml soya oil,

25 ml almond oil, 6 drops wheatgerm oil and 10 drops of the essential oil and apply to the skin directly or in a compress. Other treatments include bathing the affected skin with distilled water containing 6 drops of the essential oil, particularly a mixture of 2 drops each of lavender, juniper and cajeput. Tea tree oil can be applied directly to spots with a cotton bud, and may stop infection.

Psoriasis

The problem can be treated with aromatic oils, although the condition is very difficult to cure. Treatments include mixing together 10 ml wheatgerm oil and 2 to 3 drops of benzoin or cajeput essential oils to apply to the affected skin morning and night. Lavender oil can be used in the bath, as well as applied to the skin in a lotion or oil. A white lotion base is recommended if the psoriasis is not overdry or flaky. If the skin is very dry and the patches very scaly, an oil such as sandalwood, may be better. However, an aromatherapist should be consulted as to the exact amounts and substances to meet the needs of the individual.

Athlete's Foot

Oils that can help in the treatment of this fungal infection include tea tree, geranium and lavender. The feet can be soaked in hot water to which has been added 2 drops of the essential oil. Alternatively, a small compress with the same oils can be applied and kept in place with a cotton bandage or a sock.

Warts

Onion and garlic oils are effective and can be taken in capsule form. Raw, chopped onion and garlic applied to an overnight compress may remove warts.

Shingles

Start treatment as soon as the symptoms appear. Three drops each of geranium, sage and thyme in 20 ml carrier oil or lotion may be rubbed on to the affected area, and the same number of drops in a small glass of water may be helpful when poured on to the site or applied as a compress.

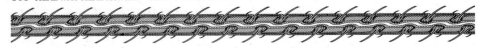

Finding A Practitioner

International Federation of Aromatherapists, 4 East Mearn Road, Dulwich, London, SE 21 8LS maintains a list of practising aromatherapists.

Further Reading

Aromatherapy by Daniele Ryman (Piatkus)
Aromatherapy: A Definitive Guide to Essential Oils by Lisa Chidell
    (Hodder & Stoughton)
Aromatherapy: Headway Lifeguides by Denise Brown
    (Hodder & Stoughton)
Aromatherapy – Massage With Essential Oils by Christine Wildwood
    (Element Books)
Massage: Headway Lifeguides by Denise Brown
    (Hodder & Stoughton)

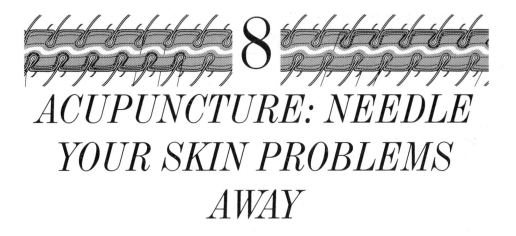

ACUPUNCTURE: NEEDLE YOUR SKIN PROBLEMS AWAY

The ancient Chinese art of acupuncture has grown in popularity in the West over the last few decades. From being considered a 'crank' therapy, it is now one of the few alternative therapies to gain widespread recognition, even by the orthodox medical profession.

The technique of inserting needles into the body to alleviate pain and to overcome disease sounds far fetched, but acupuncture's success in treating certain diseases is apparent, even if exactly how it happens is open to controversy and further research.

The technique uses very fine needles to puncture the skin at defined points along the body. This stimulates and unblocks the flow of *chi* energy, which acupuncturists believe is essential for good health.

The origins of the theory of *chi* lie in ancient China, although it is less clear as to how acupuncture was discovered. It is claimed that about 4,000 years ago, it was observed that warriors who were wounded with arrows miraculously recovered from diseases that had been troubling them for many years, prompting research with sharp needles. It was also noticed that certain organs seemed to be associated with specific points on the body which often became tender when the body was diseased, and that these points could be used for the treatment of disorders.

Original experiments were with needles made from stone, but later bone and bamboo were used. A cause-and-effect relationship was worked out by noting the point punctured and the disease it cured. When metal was discovered, the needles were made of copper, silver, gold and other alloys.

The earliest written record dates from the time of the Yellow Emperor Huang Ti, who lived in the Warring States period in China (475–221 BC), and has been reprinted in modern times as

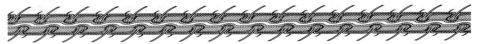

the *Yellow Emperor's Classic of Internal Medicine.*

Acupuncture was introduced into the West during the Ching dynasty (1644–1911), although the Chinese themselves attempted to ban it for political reasons. It reached Germany in the seventeenth century and then France in the middle of the nineteenth century. Due to pressure from the Western powers, which effectively ruled China at this time, the Chinese government again tried to ban traditional medicine in 1922, but its practice covertly continued until it was positively espoused by Chairman Mao in the aftermath of the Second World War, and acupuncture treatment and research was given fresh impetus and energy.

Even today, acupuncture has great grass-roots support. In China, especially, the motivation behind the development of acupuncture has been the relative poverty of the country and the lack of 'conventionally' trained physicians, drugs and medical equipment. Indeed, acupuncture is used widely by the general population, and needles and other equipment can be purchased in shops as easily as aspirin can be bought in the West.

The West's interest in acupuncture was fuelled by the writings of the French diplomat, Soulie de Morant, in the 1940s. More famously, acupuncture was brought to the attention of the West during the Presidency of Richard Nixon and 'ping-pong diplomacy' when, while visiting Peking, the renowned American commentator, James Reston, contracted acute appendicitis which required immediate surgery. This was successfully carried out under local analgesia while the postoperative pain was treated with acupuncture. This so impressed him that he visited many other centres where acupuncture was practised and, on his return to the USA, he did much to focus both professional and public attention on acupuncture.

Theory And Philosophy

In order to understand how the therapy works, it helps to have some idea of the philosophical and theoretical bases upon which acupuncture rests.

The Chinese view of the cosmos encompasses the idea that all things have a *yin* aspect and a *yang* aspect, and that without these two opposite but complementary parts, nothing could exist. So, without cold there would be no heat; without day no night. Originally, *yin* was understood to express all the qualities found on the shady side of a mountain, such as cold, wetness and darkness,

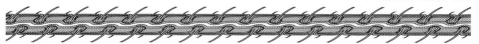

while *yang* had the qualities of the sunny side, such as heat, brightness and dryness.

Chinese philosophy also believes that all living matter is permeated by a life force or energy called *chi*. It is claimed that in the human body this energy flows along channels called *meridians*. If the body is in a state of ill health, this is because the *yin-yang* balance of the *chi* energy is upset, so that the *chi* energy is unable to flow freely. If the *yin-yang* aspects were balanced, the body would be in a state of health. So the basis of acupuncture theory is that the root cause of all disease is a problem in the energy equilibrium of the body. Treatment is concentrated on restoring this lost equilibrium.

One way of entering into the body's energy network is via the acupuncture points, of which there are about 800. These points join up to form 12 major, symmetrical meridians that are, all but one, the *triple warmer*, named after the organs to which they are attached, and are the *large intestine, stomach, heart, spleen, small intestine, bladder, circulation, kidney, gall bladder, lung, liver.* Two other meridians, the *central* and *governing*, run down the centre of the body. By manipulating the points along the meridians, it is possible to influence the *chi* and *yin-yang* balance in the organism.

How and Why Does Acupuncture Work?

The fact is, Western scientific approaches to medicine cannot explain how acupuncture works. The theory of the existence of the meridians has been questioned by a number of (mostly Western) scientists, who have found no evidence in the human body for the presence of energy channels. Yet the basic principle that problems in an organ can cause an effect or reflex to be transmitted to another part of the body, such as the skin, is generally accepted.

How the problem is remedied is another matter. One theory is that acupuncture encourages the body to release natural painkillers, such as *endorphins* and *enkephalins*, which are known to be especially beneficial in cases of depression and allergies. The painkilling effect of acupuncture is also attributed to the 'gate control' theory of pain that there are neuropathway gates to the brain via the spinal chord (if these pathways are being used by stimuli from acupuncture, they cannot be used by pain stimuli). Anaesthetic acupuncture is believed to close the gates, blocking the pain message so that we do not feel the pain, but again, this is only one part of the picture; it does not explain why acupuncture

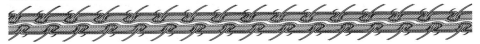

can heal non-painful conditions.

Some sceptics attribute the success of acupuncture to the placebo effect, which means that the patient, just by believing that it works, stimulates the body's own healing mechanisms, but this does not explain the long tradition of veterinary acupuncture. Others say that it is mind over matter in the same way that the power of suggestion associated with hypnosis or its state of heightened awareness stimulates physiological changes.

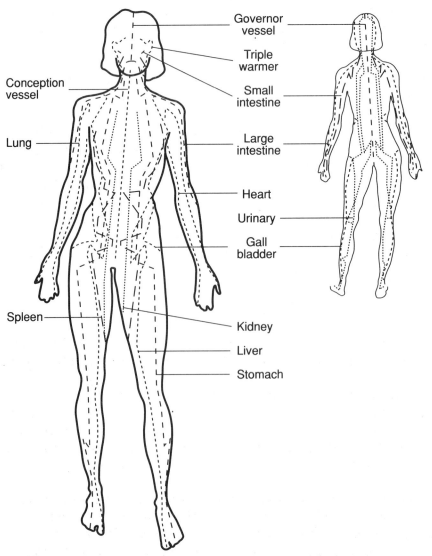

The meridians

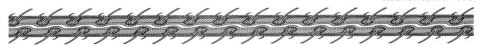

Diagnosis

In order to diagnose the patient's complaint, the acupuncturist will take a full medical history and observe particular features, such as the appearance of the face, tongue and eyes, and the condition of the skin. Aspects such as the distinctive odour of the body, personal gestures and voice tone, will assist the practitioner to make a diagnosis. Practitioners vary. Some also make a physical examination or include medical tests.

The next procedure is to check the pulses, of which there are 12, one for each meridian, six to each wrist. There are 28 qualities that can be recognised from the pulses, including tight, hasty, thin, weak, fine and slow, This technique, which takes years to master, gives the acupuncturist an insight into the gravity of the disorder and how to treat it. Pulse diagnosis is one of the main methods of determining the condition of body-energy flow.

On completion of the diagnosis, the acupuncturist decides which acupuncture points to manipulate in order to restore the balance in the patient's energy pattern. Each point has a particular function attributed to it, and it is according to this that the practitioner decides which points are to be stimulated. Often groups of points can act like a 'combination lock', i.e. their role as part of a formula is more important than their individual attributes. The most usual way to do this is with a fine needle, usually made of stainless steel.

The Use Of Needles

One's first reaction to the use of needles is usually revulsion or fear at the thought of the pain that might be felt when they are inserted into the body. Memories of painful injections or pinpricks are conjured up. But according to those who undergo acupuncture, it is a relatively painless procedure. Insertion by a skilled practitioner feels a bit like a small pinprick followed by sensation of tingling, fullness or pressure. When done correctly, it draws no blood and the sensation may be felt up to a short time afterwards.

Very fine needles are inserted obliquely, vertically or almost horizontally, usually only a fraction of an inch into the skin, although there are many other kinds of needle if specialist treatment is needed. Some needles may need to be inserted

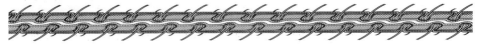

deeper into the skin, but this is not felt to be more painful than lighter insertion.

For some acupuncture treatments, a ball of dried mugwort or wormwood herb may be placed on the top of the needle's handle, inserted and set alight. A gentle heat is produced which conducts down through the needle and increases the effectiveness of the stimulation. This form of treatment is known as *moxibustion*. Some practitioners use electrical techniques whereby a device is used to produce an alternating electrical current, which is passed down the needle into the skin. Other electrical instruments may be used to detect the points which need to be stimulated, as it is known that acupuncture points are associated with decreased electrical resistance and so can be identified in this way. Electro-acupuncture is less commonly used, but may be available depending upon the practitioner. It is claimed to regulate the required energy flow with more precision and is most useful in analgesic treatment.

Another form of acupuncture, known as *auriculotherapy*, relies solely on the ear. It is based on the correlation between the ear and other parts of the body, the ear resembling the human foetus in its intrauterine position – inverted with the head pointing downwards. Two hundred points on the ear have been found for treatment. This is usually carried out by an electronic instrument that detects the points and simultaneously stimulates them, although needles are often used.

Anaesthetics And Pain Relief

Acupuncture is commonly used to alleviate pain and is sometimes used as the sole anaesthetic in China. Relief, usually for chronic pain, can be effected without the side-effects of drugs. The success of the technique depends on the nature of the problem and how far advanced it is. For acute, traumatic conditions, such as sprains and sporting injuries, pain relief through acupuncture would be a sensible initial approach. In early arthritis, acupuncture would combine well with physical treatment directed at improving mobility. However, in more chronic conditions, acupuncture might well bring little more than temporary relief. Acupuncture can help with some neuralgic pain, and alleviate the colic pains associated with gall and kidney stones. Cardiac pain, such as *angina pectoris*, may also be treated.

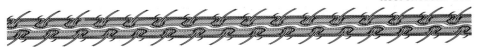

Skin Disorders

Eczema

Acupuncturists believe that eczema is associated with exposure to heat, damp and wind. The correct diagnosis and relativity of these factors can determine the success of the treatment which is based on counteracting the effects of the *pathogens* and by trying to correct any blood and energy deficiencies that might result. The meridians treated are often (although not exclusively) those corresponding to the large intestine, lungs, spleen and stomach. If the practitioner believes that the liver is not functioning properly, a special diet may be advised. Symptoms may be dealt with by applying needles to points on the hands, legs and feet. This reduces itching and inflammation of the arms and legs.

Warts

In traditional Chinese medicine, the skin is related to the lungs and the large intestine, so treatment is given to the points surrounding the warts and also to the points on the lung and large intestine meridians. Points on the governor and spleen meridians are also believed to produce anti-inflammatory and immune effects.

Shingles

Acupuncture helps to relieve the neuralgic pain associated with shingles after the initial rash has subsided. Strong manual stimulation at points on the stomach, large and small intestine and governor pain points next to the rash may also be used to relieve the pain.

Finding An Acupuncturist

The fact that anyone can call themselves acupuncturist makes it all the more important that you ascertain that the practitioner is properly trained. There are four professional bodies which are affiliated to the Council for Acupuncture, 38 Mount Pleasant, London, WC1X OAP, which maintains a register of practitioners.

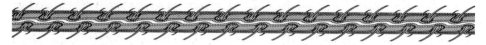

They are the British Acupuncture Association and Register, the International Register of Oriental Medicine UK, the Register of Traditional Chinese Medicine, and the Traditional Medicine Society. Before qualifying, students have to undergo a minimum three-year course which includes subjects such as anatomy, diagnosis, pathology and physiology.

Further Reading

Acupuncture by Alexander Macdonald (George Allen & Unwin)
The Acupuncture Treatment of Pain by Leon Chaitow (Thorsons)

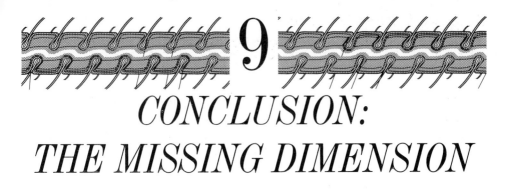

9

CONCLUSION:
THE MISSING DIMENSION

Modern man has been guided in much of his thinking by the philosopher René Descartes, whose dictum, 'I think therefore I am', crystallised his concept of dualism, of *res cognitas* (the realm of the mind) and *res extensa* (the realm of matter). His perception of the material world has so permeated our culture that we now view the human body as an elaborate machine made of assembled parts.

Descartes writes, 'I consider the human body as a machine. My thought compares the sick man and an ill-made clock with my idea of a healthy man and a well-made clock.' This legacy of reductionism has guided and moulded the basis of scientific enquiry up to the present time. The edifice of modern medicine rests on this reductionist foundation.

Modern medicine, preoccupied with measurements, statistical models and double-blind crossover studies, has focused on biological processes only, attributing the causes of all illness to biological factors. It has failed to take into account the whole person and omits to recognise the human potential for self-healing. Even the Director General of the World Health Organisation lamented that:

> Most of the world's medical schools produce doctors, not to take care of the health of people but, instead, for a medical practice that is blind to anything but disease and the technology of dealing with it; a technology involving astronomical and ever-increasing prices directed towards fewer and fewer people...

Statistics show that, despite massive investment in health care, the level of disease is rising rapidly.

Disenchantment with the high-tech, high-cost, drug-based orthodox medicine has led to a surge of interest in ancient therapies, many originating in the East. A significant proportion of GPs now refer patients to complementary therapists. The holistic model of health care has begun to gain momentum, and this has gone some way to counter the mechanistic and reductionist streaks in modern medicine.

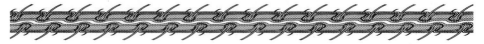

Holism believes human beings exist on more than one level, that body, mind and spirit are inextricably woven together, and that disease results from an imbalance either from within or from without. It also places its faith in the powerful and innate capacity of the body to heal itself through realignment. The primary task of the practitioner, therefore, is to encourage and assist the body in its attempts to heal itself. His or her aim is to educate rather than to intervene, and to hand back to the patient the responsibility for his or her own health.

Yet holism does not offer the complete answer, either. Holism may acknowledge the spirit 'in spirit', but this dimension often remains untouched and even avoided in practice. Without it, however, no system can be whole.

The East has taught the West that health care has many aspects not found in modern medicine. The Eastern schools of medicine, based on different world views and different cosmological principles, all have a common thread. Their principles and practices have a divine origin, and reflect our place in the universe. But are Eastern concepts really relevant to us in the West? Holistic medicine will only make sense when it is set within the framework of a world view which has a spiritual dimension. We in the West have to rediscover the concept of the divine.

The cries of holism are an inevitable reaction to the inflexibility of modern medicine. They are an expression of the dissatisfaction with the present model, and while holism may not be able to bring the divine back into the system, it can nevertheless act as a catalyst for change. Meanwhile, we need an integrated system whereby orthodox medical practitioners join hands with complementary therapists to offer the best possible system in our imperfect, spiritually-deprived society.

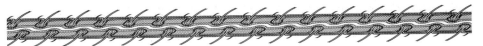

Author Profiles

Hasnain Walji is a writer and freelance journalist specialising in health, nutrition and complementary therapies, with a special interest in dietary supplementation. A contributor to several journals on environmental and Third World consumer issues, he was the founder and editor of *The Vitamin Connection – An International Journal of Nutrition, Health and Fitness,* published in the UK, Canada and Australia, focusing on the link between health and diet. He also launched Healthy Eating, a consumer magazine focusing on the concept of a well-balanced diet, and has written a script for a six-part television series, *The World of Vitamins,* shortly to be produced by a Danish Television company. His latest book, *The Vitamin Guide-Essential Nutrients for Healthy Living,* has just been published, and he is currently involved in developing NutriPlus™: a nutrition database and diet analysis programme for an American software development company.

Dr Andrea Kingston MB ChB, DRCOG, MRCGP, DCH is a Buckinghamshire GP in a five-doctor training practice who has for some years been interested in complementary approaches to healthcare as well as psychiatry and Neuro-linguistic Programming. Hypnotherapy is her major interest, and she has used this technique to help patients throughout the last eight years. As a company doctor to Volkswagen Audi, she contributes regular articles to the company magazine, *Link*. In the past, she has served as a member of the Family Practitioners Committee and as the President of the Milton Keynes Medical Society.

Books by the same authors in the Headway Healthwise series:

- Asthma & Hay Fever
- Headaches & Migraine
- Alcoholism, Smoking & Tranquillisers
- Heart Health
- Arthritis & Rheumatism

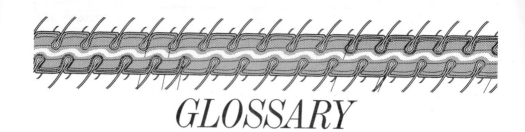

GLOSSARY

Acute Symptom that comes on suddenly, usually for a short period.

Adrenaline Hormone released by the adrenal gland, triggered by fear or stress, also called *epinephrine*.

Allergy A condition caused by the reaction of the immune system to a specific substance.

Allopathy A term used to describe conventional drug-based medicine.

Amino acids A group of chemical compounds containing nitrogen that form the basic building blocks in the production of protein. Of the 22 known amino acids, 8 are considered essential because they cannot be made by the body and therefore must be obtained from the diet.

Anaemia A condition that results when there is a low level of red blood cells.

Analgesic A substance that relieves pain.

Antibiotic A medication that helps to treat infection caused by bacteria.

Antibody Protein molecule released by the body's immune system that neutralises or counteracts foreign organism *(antigen)*.

Antidote A substance that neutralizes or counteracts the effects of a poison.

Antigen Any substance that can trigger the immune system to release an antibody to defend the body against infection and disease. When harmless substances like pollen are mistaken for harmful antigens by the immune system, allergy results.

Antihistamine A chemical that counteracts the effects of histamine, a chemical released during allergic reactions.

Antioxidants Substances which inhibit oxidation by destroying free radicals. Common antioxidants are vitamins A, C, E and the minerals selenium and zinc.

Antiseptic A preparation which has the ability to destroy undesirable microorganisms.

Artherosclerosis A disorder caused when fats are deposited in the lining of the artery wall.

Atopy A predisposition to various allergic conditions like asthma, hay fever, urticaria and eczema.

Autoimmune disease A condition in which the immune system attacks the body's own tissue e.g. rheumatoid arthritis.

Benign Non-cancerous cells; not malignant.

Beta carotene A plant substance which can be converted into vitamin A.

Bile Liquid produced in the liver for fat digestion.

Candida albicans Yeast-like fungi found in the mucous membranes of the body.

Carcinogen Cancer-causing substance or agent.

Cartilage Connective tissue that forms part of the skeletal system, such as the joints.

Chi Chinese term for the energy that circulates through the meridians.

Cholesterol A fat compound, manufactured in the body, that facilitates the transportation of fat in the blood stream.

Chronic A disorder that persists for a long time; in contrast to acute.

Cirrhosis Liver disease caused by damage of the cells and internal scarring (*fibrosis*).

Collagen Main component of the connective tissue.

Constitutional treatment Treatment determined by an assessment of a person's physical, mental and emotional states.

Contagious A term referring to a disease that can be transferred from one person to another by direct contact.

Corticosteroid Drugs used to treat inflammation similar to corticosteroid hormones produced by the adrenal glands that control the body's use of nutrients and excretion of salts and water in urine.

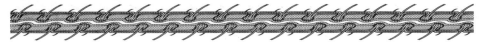

Detoxification   Treatment to eliminate or reduce poisonous substances *(toxins)* from the body.

Diuretic   Substance that increases urine flow.

DNA   A molecule carrying genetic information in most organisms.

Elimination diet   A diet which eliminates allergic foods.

Endorphins   Substances which have the property of suppressing pain. They are also involved in controlling the body's response to stress.

Enzyme   A protein catalyst that speeds chemical reactions in the body.

Essential fatty acids   Substances that cannot be made by the body and therefore need to be obtained from the diet.

Free radicals   Highly unstable atom or group of atoms that can bind to and

Hepatic   Pertaining to the liver.

Histamine   A chemical released during an allergic reaction, responsible for redness and swelling that occur in inflammation.

Holistic medicine   Any form of therapy aimed at treating the whole person – mind, body and spirit.

Keratin   A protein found in the outermost layer of the skin, nails and hair.

Lymphocyte   A type of white blood cell found in lymph nodes. Some lymphocytes are important in the immune system.

Malignant   A term that describes a condition that gets progressively worse resulting in death.

Melanoma, malignant   A form of skin cancer.

Mast cell   A cell that secretes histamine and other inflammatory chemicals and plays an important part in allergy.

Meridian   Energy pathways that connect the acupuncture and acupressure points and the internal organs.

Mucous membrane   Pink tissue that lines most cavities and tubes in the body, such as the mouth, nose etc.

Mucus   The thick fluid secreted by the mucous membranes.

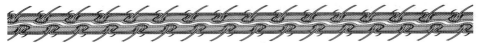

Neurotransmitter A chemical that transmits nerve impulses between nerve cells.

Oxidation Chemical process of combining with oxygen or of removing hydrogen.

Placebo A chemically inactive substance given instead of a drug, often used to compare the efficacy of medicines in clinical trials.

Potency A term used in homoeopathy to describe the number of times a substance has been diluted.

Prostaglandin Hormone-like compounds manufactured from essential fatty acids.

Sclerosis Process of hardening or scarring.

Stimulant A substance that increases energy.

Toxin A poisonous protein produced by disease-causing bacteria.

Vaccine A preparation given to induce immunity against a specific infectious disease.

Vasoconstriction A term used to describe the constriction of blood vessels.

Vitamin Essential nutrient that the body needs to act as a catalyst in normal processes of the body.

Withdrawal Termination of a habit-forming substance.

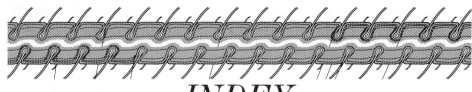

INDEX

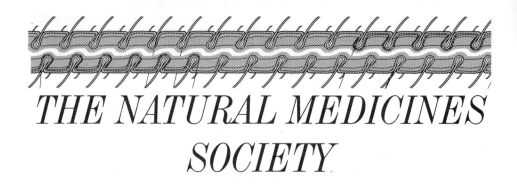

THE NATURAL MEDICINES SOCIETY

The Natural Medicines Society is a registered charity representing the consumer voice for freedom of choice in medicine. The Society needs the support of every individual who uses natural medicines and who is concerned about their continued existence in order to achieve the necessary changes needed to accomplish their wider availability and acceptance within the NHS.

The Society's aims are to improve the standing and practice of natural medicine by encouraging education and research, and by co-operating with the government and the EC on their registration, safety and efficacy. A major drawback in this work has been that none of the Department of Health's licensing bodies has any experts from these systems of medicine sitting on their committees – this has meant that not one of the natural medicines assessed by them has been judged by anyone with an understanding of the therapy's practice. Since the formation of the Society, it has worked towards the establishment of expert representation on the committees appraising these medicines.

To fulfil these aims, the NMS formed the Medicines Advisory Research Committee in February 1988. Known as MARC, its members are doctors, practitioners, pharmacists and other experts in natural medicines. It is the members of MARC who undertake much of the necessary technical and legal work. They have discussed and submitted proposals to the Department of Health's Medicines Control Agency (MCA), on how the EC Directive for Homoeopathic Medicinal Products can be incorporated into the existing UK system, and how medicines outside the orthodox range can be fairly evaluated.

The EC Directive for Homoeopathic Medicinal Products was eventually passed as European law in September 1992, incorporating anthroposophical and biochemic medicines, as well as homoeopathic. With discussions regarding the implementation of the Homoeopathic Directive now in progress, the MARC's work

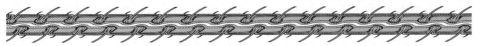

begins in earnest.

In July 1993, the MCA sent out their consultation paper regarding the implementation of the Directive, which incorporates many of the suggestions submitted by MARC. In it they propose to set up a committee of experts to advise on the registration of homoeopathic, anthroposophic and biochemic medicines. This is a major step forward for the Society, and homoeopathy in general.

With MARC members becoming increasingly involved in the legislative process of the implementation of the Directive, the Natural Medicines Society can now move forward from the short-term aim of protecting the availability of the medicines, to the longer-term aims of promoting and developing their usage and status by instigating and supporting research and education. The NMS has already sponsored some research – it is important to stress here that the Society does not endorse, support or condone animal experimentation – including an expedition to the rain forests in search of medicinal plants, supporting a cancer research project at the Royal London Homoeopathic Hospital and contributing to a methodology Research Fellowship. On the educational side, the Society has published two booklets, with several more planned and has co-sponsored a seminar for doctors and medical students.

The Natural Medicines Society depends upon its membership to continue this unique and important work – please add your support by joining us.

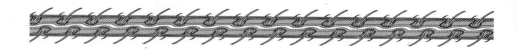

IF YOU ARE NOT ALREADY A MEMBER WHY NOT JOIN THE NATURAL MEDICINES SOCIETY?

Mr/Mrs/Miss/Ms _____ (BLOCK CAPITALS PLEASE)

Address _____

_____

Postcode _____ Tel. No. _____

There is no 'fixed' annual membership fee. Please indicate below the amount you wish to pay: minimum £5 (students and unwaged); European countries £15; non-EC £20.

£5 _____ £10 _____ £15 _____

N.B. Pay by Deed of Covenant and/or Direct Debit if you can—please ask for details.

Donations and offers of practical help are also always welcome to aid our fight to return natural medicines to the mainstream of medical practice.

I enclose a donation of £ _____

Please return this form with your remittance (cheques and PO's payable to The Natural Medicines Society), to:

THE NMS MEMBERSHIP OFFICE,
EDITH LEWIS HOUSE,
ILKESTON,
DERBYS,
DE7 8EJ.

(Registered charity no.327468)

You will receive your Membership Card, Member's Handbook, Quarterly Newsletter.